Advance Praise for
The Stutter Steps

"Sander's book is not only instructional, it is inspirational. In telling his own story and that of so many other stutterers while coupling it with an array of advice, this book combines what is so desperately needed—sound counsel and emotional support."

—**Michael Sheehan**, Sheehan Associates

"A book that provides an important window into this mysterious challenge. Stuttering is deeply personal for Sander, and he symbolizes the courage to speak freely and live fearlessly."

—**Aaron Graff**, Executive Vice President, Chief Commercial Officer,
Ferring Pharmaceuticals

"Sander Flaum's friendship and support over the years has been an inspiration to me as a fellow stutterer. In this book he communicates the anguish of this genetic condition as he offers a better understanding of stuttering to those who don't, and potential treatment solutions to those who do."

—**Michael Conforti**, Director Emeritus, Clark Art Institute;
Adjunct Professor, Williams College

"Good advice! Wish I'd had the guts to 'go ahead and stutter.' Hiding my stutter hurt me more than my stuttering ever did."

—**John Stossel**, TV Anchor

"Sander Flaum's most recent book is a special gift to the over 70 million people in the world who are challenged by stuttering. His thoughtful and engaging way of dealing with the subject will give encouragement not only to those of us with speech disorders but also to those interested in moving beyond the many myths associated with this misunderstood affliction."

—**Susan Reichardt**, Ph.D.

"By embracing the importance of accepting yourself for who you are, Sander offers the reader the encouragement and inspiration needed to speak freely and live fearlessly. He dives deeply into the latest therapeutic approaches to stuttering treatment and provides real-life examples of how successful individuals learned to use their stuttering as a source of strength. *The Stutter Steps* is an excellent resource for those looking to gain confidence and communicate more effectively."

—**Nolan Russo Jr.**, Vice President, Business Development, Capital Printing

"Sander is a mentor and model for me. What he has achieved in his professional and personal life is remarkable, and his tireless efforts on behalf of the American Institute for Stuttering inspired me to follow in his footsteps as the newest Chair. The Institute and the stuttering community are meaningfully better off because of Sander, and we will always be grateful."

—**Eric Dinallo**, Chair of Insurance Regulatory Practice at Debevoise & Plimpton LLP

"*The Stutter Steps* should be must-reading for everyone afflicted with this speech disorder and their loved ones—especially for its messages that you're not alone, and that highly effective therapy is available."

—**Alan Tonelson**, Founder, RealtyChek, a public policy blog

THE STUTTER STEPS

PROVEN PATHWAYS
TO SPEAKING CONFIDENTLY
AND LIVING COURAGEOUSLY

SANDER A. FLAUM

WITH WES SMITH

Post Hill
PRESS

A POST HILL PRESS BOOK

The Stutter Steps:
Proven Pathways to Speaking Confidently and Living Courageously
© 2021 by Sander A. Flaum
All Rights Reserved

ISBN: 978-1-64293-653-7
ISBN (eBook): 978-1-64293-654-4

Cover art by Cody Corcoran
Interior design and composition by Greg Johnson, Textbook Perfect

Post Hill Press
New York • Nashville
posthillpress.com

Published in the United States of America
1 2 3 4 5 6 7 8 9 10

This book is dedicated to my beautiful and late wife,
Mechele, who died in November 2017.
We had a wonderful life together.
She was inspiring, supportive,
and the most loving person I have ever known.
May she rest in peace.

CONTENTS

FOREWORD

By Dr. Heather Grossman, PhD, CCC-SLP, BCS-F,
Director of the American Institute for Stuttering

My career as a speech-language pathologist began in the late 1980s. At the time, most of the therapy techniques for both children and adults who stuttered focused on physical "tools" that were intended to eliminate the person's stutter.

I quickly noticed, however, that while these therapy techniques did indeed increase fluency to a certain degree, many of my clients could not successfully utilize them in the situations where they most desired fluency.

The training I had received in graduate school was largely focused on the physical components of stuttering. Within the therapy session, we would present clients with tools such as easy onsets, light articulatory contacts, pausing, and so on. We would then work on transferring the skills by taking clients to talk in stores and restaurants.

While "counseling" was considered an important part of the therapeutic process, we were inadequately trained for that aspect of treatment. What most therapists were calling counseling actually amounted to little more than talking through the personal challenges of transferring fluency skills.

Not only did clients find it difficult to use their tools consistently, many commented that they did not *like* the way they sounded using the tools. A large proportion found that in high-stress situations, their fluency skills would "fly out the window."

I did not understand this dynamic at the time, but we now know that when a person who stutters enters a highly feared situation, a fight or flight response can kick in. In this state, the body's physiological tension is sky-high. The ability to engage higher cognitive centers is lost. It started to make more and more sense that the fear of stuttering and speaking could render many speech tools useless.

Dedicated to learning as much as I could about stuttering, I immersed myself in the stuttering self-help community. I spent a lot of time listening. When I first attended the annual conference of the National Stuttering Association (at the time, the National Stuttering Project), I was quite shocked at the intensity of animosity directed toward speech-language pathologists. I learned that many people felt that their lack of success achieving and/or maintaining fluency through speech therapy created a secondary cycle of hopelessness, shame, and guilt, which only made their stuttering *worse*, ultimately.

I realized that we needed to approach stuttering from an entirely new perspective. In addition to the invaluable education I received from people who stutter and attending self-help conferences, I returned to graduate school in 2005. There, I attained my PhD. My thesis was on the phenomenon of voluntary stuttering.

I learned to approach stuttering from a client-driven perspective, while recognizing the many variables that contribute to each individual's unique stuttering profile. I immersed myself in exploring Rational Emotive Behavior Therapy as a way to help people who stutter. This approach targets the unhelpful core beliefs that people who stutter tend to hold about themselves and their speech.

I met Sander Flaum in 2011 when I was transitioning into my position as director of the American Institute for Stuttering in NYC. Sander was chairman of the AIS Board of Directors at that time. I had already completed the formal interview process and was to begin in August of that year.

I received a call from Sander one afternoon, intended simply as an introduction and welcome. Besides his obvious warmth and friendly demeanor, I was struck by his openness about my approach to stuttering treatment.

I knew Sander had great success with the Hollins program many years earlier. Given that I had some very strong reservations about that approach, I was frankly concerned that Sander would expect me to follow a fluency shaping philosophy at AIS.

True philanthropy involves helping people and not promoting causes, and I came to learn that Sander is a true philanthropist. Despite his personal success following a fluency shaping approach, he generously supports those seeking quite different approaches.

Clinic areas at both the Ohio State University and the American Institute for Stuttering have been named in his honor, reflecting his ongoing support helping individuals who stutter. His impetus in writing this book emanates from a desire to provide inspiration, hope, and encouragement—especially to those who have feelings of isolation and hopelessness because of their stuttering.

When I was supervising graduate student interns back in the early nineties, people who stutter were admitted into graduate programs. However, in order to pass their clinical internships, it was generally expected that those students would speak fluently during their assessments and treatment.

I found it disturbing that many students were told they would not be allowed to graduate if they were not "fluent enough" during their internships. Well, cut to 2020 and I am proud to report that many of the most effective, talented therapists I know are people who stutter—and continue to stutter with varying degrees of frequency and tension.

Today, stuttering research is driven by people such as Naomi Rogers, Michael Boyle, Chris Constantino, and Caryn Herring. All of them stutter and understand the complexities and nuances of stuttering.

There is most definitely a new generation of people who stutter. They have overcome the shackles of stuttering and are dedicated to the opposite of "old-school avoidance." Rather than try to hide stuttering, they self-disclose with confidence. They advocate for themselves and for all who stutter. They speak (and stutter) openly. The very notion of how we should view stuttering is being called into question. One alternative might be to view stuttering as similar to a "foreign accent."

The worldview of stuttering is shifting, but there is still a lot to do. Unfortunately, there is still a great deal of public misunderstanding regarding stuttering.

This book will introduce you to many people who have successfully learned to live free of the self-limiting confines of their stuttering. Many of these individuals continue to stutter in varying degrees. That is important, because we often infer that someone who has "overcome" stuttering no longer stutters, which is not always true.

When we speak of someone who has "overcome stuttering," therapists mean that stuttering no longer dictates their life choices or holds them back from what they want to say or what they want to do. They no longer experience the anticipatory dread that had once preceded speaking situations, nor do they feel the shame that habitually accompanied episodes of severe stuttering.

In Sander's book, you will read about some extraordinary people, and their various paths to becoming confident, effective communicators, with or without stuttering. Those who stutter define their own success in very different ways, and therefore, progress looks quite different for different people.

I am proud to know many of the individuals in the following chapters, and am excited Sander has presented their stories to illustrate that there truly is no one-size-fits-all approach to stuttering treatment.

If you do not stutter, you will likely be surprised to learn how dramatically stuttering has impacted the lives of some very well-known individuals who you probably never knew stuttered. If you stutter and continue to feel held back by fear, self-doubt, and struggles related to your speech, you will be encouraged to learn that even if you feel you have tried it all, it is never too late to open up and try something new.

As someone who has seen thousands of others succeed, I encourage you to keep your mind, heart, and eyes open to the very real possibility that you too will find a path to freeing your voice and speaking your mind.

1

Speak with Ease and Live with Confidence!

"*Because you have a stammer, you'll always have to work harder and be smarter than the competition.*"

My wonderful mother and mentor, Rose Flaum, offered that advice many times throughout my life to encourage me in dealing with my speaking challenges, which made me the subject of taunts and harsh judgments both in childhood and even into adulthood.

My nose was broken twice in fights that I initiated after being mocked for my stuttering. Others tried to break my spirit more times than I can count.

Let's just say I was better at protecting my spirit than my nose. The goal of this book is to help you protect your spirit, too. In fact, the information and stories in this book will lift your morale, your confidence, your self-assurance, and your heart.

Many of those who stutter feel frustrated because there are so many theories about the cause of stuttering. They wonder if it is a physical issue, a psychological problem, or something else altogether. That is understandable, because even speech pathologists and therapists are still searching for answers. They know more than they did when I first sought treatment more than fifty years ago, but it's been hard to come up with any definitive answers.

There is now a growing belief that stuttering is rooted in genetics. For example, the actress Emily Blunt, who stutters and serves on the American Institute for Stuttering (AIS) Board of Directors, notes that her uncle, cousin, and grandfather also stuttered.

Additionally, there are neurological and physiological causes to stuttering. Some sort of weakness in linguistic encoding along with motor production may be associated with stuttering onset. There may be emotional factors as well. The experts will tell you that the problem of stuttering in school children and adults often is due to coping strategies that those of us who stutter learn in order to deal with stuttering.

People who stutter (like me) tend to avoid eye contact, words that trip us up, and social settings where we might have to talk to strangers. We do whatever we can, including the use of filler sounds such as "um" and "ah," to get through our stuttering. Those avoidance methods become habits.

The psychological aspects stem from our efforts to avoid negative reactions, as well as the shame, embarrassment, and frustrations we feel. This component leads us to self-defeating thoughts and actions, like turning down promotions for jobs that require more face-to-face meetings with co-workers or clients.

According to the Stuttering Foundation of America, 1 percent of the population stutters, and four times as many males as females stutter. You will read in these pages many, many stories of other men, women, and children who have built wonderful lives for themselves—even though they too have speaking challenges because of stuttering.

Some of these people are famous celebrities, like the singer Ed Sheeran and the aforementioned actress Emily Blunt, whose names you see and hear all the time. Some are successful business-people who've built or lead multi-million-dollar companies and organizations.

Some have even served in the White House, like former vice president Joe Biden. Biden talked openly during the 2020 presidential campaign about his lifelong struggle with stuttering, which he still deals with, especially when working long hours on the campaign trail. "It has nothing to do with your intelligence quotient. It has nothing to do with your intellectual makeup," he said during a CNN town hall appearance. Biden said he stays in touch with about fifteen others who stutter. They encourage each other, and he tells them it is "critically important for them not to judge themselves by their speech—and to not let that define them."

At an earlier appearance on the campaign trail, Biden met a father and his twelve-year-old son who stutters. The father asked the former vice president for guidance and they talked privately a little later. In that discussion, Biden said his own mother would tell him, "Joey, don't let this define you. Joey, remember who you are. Joey, you can do it," according to a CNN report on their meeting.

Biden's honesty about stuttering and his encouragement is important, because there are many more regular people like you and me who don't make headlines or millions of dollars—but we still enjoy our lives and careers, because we've found ways to overcome or manage our stutter so we can go out and chase our dreams.

As I noted, I have stuttered all my life, and I continue to stutter even now as a "senior citizen" and grandfather. With the help of my mother and many speech therapists and experts—as well as some methods I've devised myself—I've had success in a number of career fields. Still, I understand that does not make me a true expert on this topic.

I've tapped into the true experts at AIS, where I served as the former chairman of the board of directors, and at Dr. Ronald Webster's Hollins Communications Research Institute (HCRI), where I underwent speech therapy in the 1960s.

Thanks, in particular, to the professionals at AIS, this book will offer you a wide range of proven therapies and techniques for overcoming stuttering. Please, as you read through each chapter, keep in mind that at AIS, in particular, most clients benefit from not just one therapeutic approach, but a combination that might include changing to more positive thoughts, voluntary stuttering, self-help programs, self-disclosure of stuttering, and public speaking. My goal is to tell you about each therapy so that you understand the options available to you based on your goals.

AIS is a not-for-profit center founded in 1998 by a beloved and respected speech therapist, the late Catherine Otto Montgomery. AIS provides state-of-the-art speech therapy to people who stutter. They do this in their headquarters in New York and Atlanta, and through online courses accessible to nearly anyone.

This terrific organization also offers guidance to families and clinical training to speech professionals. The folks at AIS are activists, too. They serve as a powerful voice, one that calls for government support of stuttering research and legislation.

I am proud that AIS and HCRI have helped tens of thousands of people who stutter find paths to better lives. AIS surveys have shown that 98 percent of the people who they work with believe that their lives are better as a result.

As this book makes clear, there is no one sure cure for stuttering—no magic pill—but the therapeutic approaches have come a long way and continue to improve. The truth is that there are now a number of methods for helping those with stutters, and, as I will note throughout the book, often it is a combination of these methods that works best. It just depends on the person.

That is another important point made in this book: every person who stutters is unique, and the methods that can help them may not be the same as those that have helped others.

As AIS Director Dr. Heather Grossman, who kindly wrote the foreword for this book and served as a generous resource, sharing her expertise and knowledge, is fond of reminding me, "Different people have found success in quite different ways."

You Decide What Works Best for YOU!

Please note that this book isn't about telling you what to do. It's about helping you figure out what works best for you—and encouraging you to never give up, but instead to speak freely and live fearlessly. Many people who stutter have found or created their own successful methods for overcoming their challenges.

The singer Ed Sheeran, for example, told us in AIS gatherings that his stuttering diminished over time after he began rapping along with Eminem! Can you believe that? Speech therapist experts at AIS have told me that there is an important lesson to be learned in this wonderful and inspiring story. When Ed rapped to Eminem's recordings, he enjoyed himself so much that he no longer allowed his stutter to dominate his thoughts, or his image of himself. Feel free to try the Ed Sheeran "Eminem Method" and see if it works for you.

"Be yourself, embrace your quirks, being weird is a wonderful thing, and it has been for so many creative people," he said in a speech at an AIS benefit in 2015. "No one can be a better you than you."

The big lesson in his success story is that overcoming the fear of stuttering can be a very helpful step toward reducing or eliminating stuttering itself. Though it should be noted that a change in perspective does not guarantee any adjustments occurring in your speech.

As I've mentioned, experts definitely feel there are genetic reasons most people stutter. They also believe stuttering becomes more severe and can be aggravated by the negative emotions and thoughts that develop over time, especially if the person was teased as a child, like me and so many others.

The AIS therapy team says many people who come to them for help are "covert" in their stuttering. They typically do not stutter in normal conversation, but they live with intense anxiety that they *might* stutter. Those who hide their stutters tend to avoid certain words, self-edit their speech, and use tricks they've devised to hide their stuttering.

The more serious issue is that this group of people who stutter covertly often put limits on themselves and their lives because of their fear of stuttering. They may turn down promotions, skip social events, and isolate themselves at work or socially. This book will offer them special guidance for dealing with their fears, because I believe everyone deserves the best possible life.

As you read this book, keep in mind that while there are now many different approaches to relieve anxiety and improve speech fluency for people who stutter, most derive the greatest benefits from customized therapy plans that include several different methods and ideologies.

There are different methods available to you, just as there are different ways to define success for those who stutter. I know people who still have difficulty with fluid speech, but they consider themselves successful because they have greatly reduced their fear of speaking and become more comfortable communicating. Some people, when they leave a treatment program, actually stutter more…but they feel great about what they've accomplished because they have conquered their fear. They've learned to speak without feeling like they are treading through a minefield.

As many of us know, stuttering can take away the spontaneity of speaking freely. The goal is to ease the fear of stuttering so you don't worry about it, and can just think about *what* you are saying rather than *how* you are saying it. Making that shift alone can be a great boost.

My goal with this book is to help you understand all of the approaches. I want you to be open to trying anything and everything that you think might work for you.

Key Component: Accept Yourself!
You Don't Have to be Perfect All the Time

While there is no one surefire cure for stuttering, the vast majority of those who have overcome its challenges do have one thing in common: they've learned to accept themselves and love themselves, which opens the door for others to accept and love them too. Once you learn to do that, you will find that your fear and anxiety over stuttering is greatly diminished.

You may not stop stuttering completely or forever, but so what? You may stutter, but your stutter does not define you! And guess what? Many of the people who stutter I've known actually believe that stuttering has helped make them a more compassionate, interesting, and determined person.

Many of the celebrities and regular people featured in this book will tell you that they still stutter sometimes, but they don't let it bother them. *You don't have to be perfect!* Say that to yourself and you will immediately feel a burden lifted. You can choose to let go of perfection, accept yourself, and still be the best you can be. I've seen this work for people from all walks of life.

Award-winning actor Samuel L. Jackson, who stutters, learned to do this even in school. When other kids made fun of his speaking challenges, he used their teasing as motivation to be a top student, and then a highly acclaimed performer. He still uses that method today. The actor who has appeared in *Star Wars* prequels as well as *Iron Man, The Avengers, Pulp Fiction,* and *Jurassic Park,* said that while filming *Captain America,* when the director yelled, "Action!" he stuttered his first line and it came out "G-g-g-et."

Samuel didn't freak out. Instead, he laughed to himself and said, "I guess I'm having a '*g-g-g* day.' Sometimes I have '*p-p-p* days' or '*b-b-b* days.' I'm still stuttering, but I have figured out a way to do it."

Samuel, who has been listed as the highest-grossing actor of all time, didn't feel bad about himself. He laughed it off and just rolled with it. You can learn to do the same.

My promise is that this book will provide guidance to help you on your path to greater self-confidence and more free-flowing speech fluency, whether you continue to stutter or not. The goal is to open your eyes to ways that allow you to communicate more effectively, to be comfortable stuttering and talking about stuttering, to remain confident and self-assured even when you do stutter, and to feel free to speak without any fear or shame.

"Speak Freely, Live Fearlessly" is the motto of the AIS, and I believe everyone who stutters should adopt that same positive and encouraging goal. All of those who stutter have to find ways to overcome adversity. I know this as someone who has stuttered throughout my life. I've fought the good fight and I'm still fighting it today. I want to encourage you in this book, the same way my mother encouraged me when she said, "You always have a choice when you run into a major challenge."

We do have that choice. We may not speak as fluently as we'd like, but that doesn't mean we can't build successful and happy lives. But you don't have to take it from me. In this book I will provide you with scores of examples of men, women, and children who have made the choice to never let their stuttering define them or limit their lives.

I will also tell you about regular people who've built extraordinary lives, and even some who've risen to the very top of their fields. Did you know, for example, that the late Jack Welch—the respected former CEO of General Electric—once left that remarkable company because someone told him that his stuttering would hinder his career? Or that the co-founder of Home Depot, Arthur Blank, rose above his stuttering to build one of the most successful retail companies of modern times?

You have probably watched movies starring Emily Blunt, Bruce Willis, and Samuel L. Jackson without realizing that, like you, they have stuttered throughout their lives. Others include singers Carly Simon and the late Bill Withers, whose songs are heard around the world.

They are all fighting the good fight like you and me. They don't let their speaking challenges limit their lives. Instead, they are determined to focus on developing their minds and their talents. They build on their strengths to overcome any challenges.

I have met hundreds of—maybe a thousand—people who've made the choice to control their own destinies without limits, despite their speaking challenges. They've done it. I've done it. You can do it too, and in this book, you will find the information, tools, and encouragement to pursue your dreams. I will show you the path to your best life.

To reiterate, however, please understand there is not a one-size-fits-all approach to stuttering treatment. So, in this book we will look at a variety of methods, techniques, approaches, mindsets, and combinations of these elements.

I will offer information on:

- Avoidance reduction and stuttering for a purpose
- Stuttering modification therapy
- Self-advertising your stuttering
- Fluency shaping
- Mindfulness and meditation
- Holistic approaches
- Public speaking as stuttering therapy
- Creative passions to manage stuttering
- Support groups and networks
- Parental guidance for children who stutter

Each of us can find a path according to our unique abilities and needs. The experts will tell you that stuttering is linked to our genes, but they will also tell you that there are many ways we can overcome our fears, frustrations, and anxieties over it.

For most of those who stutter—and also those who treat them—the goal is fluency in speech and a lack of fear, anxiety, and shame. But you should also be aware of an interesting new wave in this field that promotes "stuttering pride."

At the forefront of this wave is Chris Constantino, PhD, a highly respected speech-language pathologist and assistant professor at Florida State University. Along with teaching classes on counseling and stuttering, he conducts extensive research on the subjective experience of stuttering and how it interacts with culture and society.

Regarded as a leading-edge thinker in his field, Dr. Constantino, who stutters himself, challenges the stereotype that stuttering is inherently negative. He maintains that it is a different, valuable, and respected way of speaking, a philosophy reflected in the book *Stammering Pride and Prejudice: Difference Not Defect*, which he co-edited.

Dr. Constantino suggests that those who stutter should celebrate and take pride in their speech disability so that it is no longer seen as a negative, or as the opposite of fluency. He has taken part in many programs and discussions at AIS, making the case that there are positives to stuttering even though society tends to discriminate against those with speech disabilities.

"There are many, many people who still take the stance that fluency of speech is the best for those who stutter. But there is a growing dialogue about the depth of human connection that stuttering can bring to communications, which could not exist between fluent speakers," AIS Director Heather Grossman told me while I was researching this book. "Chris is a leader in this modern wave that encourages people who stutter to take pride in the disability, not just by talking about it, but showing it."

This new approach contends that stuttering is a different way of communicating, but still legitimate and not merely "a less fluent" way of communicating. Dr. Constantino promotes the idea that stuttering adds to our speech rather than detracting from it.

"The irregular rhythms of our speech allow for open and honest communication unburdened by meaningless, stereotyped phrases. When people speak to us, it breaks them out of their routine," he wrote in a 2016 paper for the International Stuttering Association entitled "Stuttering Gain."

This theory holds that others listen to those who stutter more closely because they are less predictable, which makes conversations with them more interesting and memorable.

"Just by saying hello, we deeply connect with another person," Dr. Constantino wrote in "Stuttering Gain." "Every moment of stuttering is an exercise in trust, a verbal trust fall. We are asking the person we are speaking with to catch us. When they do, we build trust and strengthen the relationship.... The reward of stuttering and being heard is a deeply intimate connection with another human being. I encourage us to take this risk."

This is an approach that I'd never considered, but I believe it is worth sharing.

In fact, most speech therapists agree that your focus should be on self-acceptance and self-determination more than recovery or finding a complete cure. Many high-achieving people will tell you that they still stutter now and then. Some even stutter more than ever. But their stuttering does not slow them down or limit their opportunities.

As I was writing this book, I was surprised to see a guest editorial about overcoming stuttering in the *New York Times*. It was written by a famous individual, a hero really, whom I'd never known to stutter, even though I'd heard him speak many times. They even made a movie with Tom Hanks portraying him.

His name is Chesley "Sully" Sullenberger, and he was the "Captain Sully" airline pilot who won the praise and admiration of the world when he managed to safely land a full commercial passenger plane that had lost all power in the Hudson River of New York City.

In his *New York Times* opinion piece, Capt. Sullenberger wrote that as a boy growing up in Texas, he anguished over being called on in class. He would flush with fear because of concerns that his words "could not keep up with [his] mind, and they would come out jumbled."

He suffered humiliation and bullying because of the "inability to get the words out," he wrote.

Captain Sullenberger said memories of those feelings returned when a member of President Trump's family mocked Joe Biden's stuttering at a Trump campaign event by saying, "Joe, can you get it out?"

The famed pilot wrote that similar bullying had caused "childhood agony," and in his article, he implored people to stop taunting those who stutter. Capt. Sullenberger explained that over time, he learned to manage and overcome his stuttering by slowing down his speech and enunciating each word carefully. He also found that singing in the church choir helped him to control his breathing and word formation.

"I learned to resist and overcome the bullying," he wrote. "I also learned that our imperfections do not define us."

As he noted in his *New York Times* article, Capt. Sullenberger went on to a successful career as a U.S. Air Force fighter pilot, an airline pilot, and a public speaker. In a moving passage, he wrote that when a bird strike knocked out both engines of his US Airways passenger plane in January 2009 and he announced his plan to conduct an emergency landing in the Hudson River, "my words came out with precision and control, even in the stress of a life-threatening emergency."

Capt. Sully ended his poignant piece by offering encouragement to children and others who stutter, noting that "a speech disorder is a lot easier to treat than a character defect." The veteran pilot went on to say:

> *You are fine, just as you are. You can do any job you dream of when you grow up. Ignore kids (and adults) who are mean, or don't know what it feels like to stutter. Respond by showing them how to be kind, polite, respectful and generous, to be brave enough to try big things, even though you are not perfect.*

Most of us thought Capt. Sully was a hero because he saved so many lives when he skillfully landed his passenger plane on the river. But with this article, we learned that he has always been a heroic person.

From all of us who have struggled and strived to overcome our stuttering, just like you, thank you, Capt. Sully!

2

Avoidance Reduction Therapy and Stuttering for a Purpose

Chaya Goldstein often writes on the AIS website and talks at AIS events about the many years she spent as a "master avoider." She tried to hide the fact that she stuttered, fearing that she would be discovered.

"I avoided people, places, conversation, and opportunities. I was tagged 'the quiet one,' 'mysterious,' and the 'best listener.' No one knew how I hated those titles, or just how much I had to say," she wrote in an AIS website essay called "My Journey Home."

She said her closeted life as someone who covertly stuttered was exhausting and took its toll. Finally, at the age of nineteen, she decided to face her stuttering head on.

"I knew in my heart this path would lead me to the light," she wrote. "It was the only way to go."

Instead of avoiding her stutter, she went after it with a vengeance. She signed up for college classes on the fundamentals of speech and language to learn everything she could about human communication.

Diving in deeper, she took a three-week internship at AIS in New York City. There, Chaya worked as a student clinician and found herself asking clients to do things she had never dared to do herself, including voluntary stuttering, advertising or announcing your stutter, and exploring moments of stuttering.

"Terrified, I realized I had arrived," she recalled. "I made a commitment to step into the experience fully. With my clients, I blazed the path of uncertainty and bravery, embracing the ups and downs of stuttering and exploring the complexities and range of experiences stuttering brings."

By the end of her internship, she decided to enroll in the AIS intensive program the following summer. She faced her fears during that experience and emerged feeling free and ready to take on the world.

"I owned my stutter and ran with it," she noted. "It was terrifying, overwhelming, exhilarating and empowering all at the same time."

She had found a home at AIS, quite literally. Today, Chaya is a speech-language pathologist in the AIS New York office, where she has a passion for helping others find their power and joy in communicating. She co-leads the Manhattan chapter of the National Stuttering Association, teaches graduate classes on stuttering and fluency disorders, and is a passionate advocate for those who stutter, whether it is in schools, work environments, or healthcare settings.

"Today I continue to walk forth with my mission: supporting others in discovering their voice and celebrating the freedom that comes from living fearlessly and speaking freely," Chaya says.

Avoidance Methods

These are typical avoidance tactics for those of us who stutter:

- Avoiding eye contact while stuttering and speaking to others
- Replacing words with those that don't trip you up
- Saying filler words such as "um" or "ah" before difficult words
- Letting the phone ring rather than picking it up
- Skipping social gatherings or remaining on the sidelines rather than speaking to people
- Texting rather than calling, even when you want to talk with someone
- Using gestures and other physical movements to get your words out

Avoidance reduction therapy focuses on easing the interior conflicts and fears that drive us to do all of the above. Speech therapists believe that attempts to avoid or hide stuttering really only make it worse in the long run, and often in the short run too.

This approach often includes having conversations with your clinician about daily life, and particularly about recent times when you've felt more comfortable in speaking with others.

Sessions applying avoidance reduction therapy often include discussions with the speech therapist about situations that make you anxious or fearful, as well as developing a plan for reducing those negative feelings by stuttering voluntarily or using other methods. Your speech therapist might suggest you make a specific number of phone calls each day to help you become more comfortable with speaking. You might be encouraged to speak more freely and keep eye contact as you talk with people you feel safe with, like family members or friendly co-workers.

Like many who stutter, Chaya had adopted avoidance behaviors—such as limiting her communication with others, avoiding situations where she might have to speak, and substituting words that triggered her stutter. Unfortunately, even though these avoidances seem to eliminate some stuttering, they only serve to increase fear and perpetuate more avoidance for those of us who stutter, according to many speech therapists.

Then, when we stutter despite our best efforts to avoid it, our bodies tense up. Often, our stuttering is most severe when we are trying our best to be fluent.

And so, this is why the team at AIS encourages their clients to avoid avoidance, or to at least cut back on their efforts to avoid stuttering as at least one aspect of their therapy: "The core of the problem of stuttering is actually made up of all the things the person does in order *not* to stutter," Dr. Grossman says. "We find that once individuals accept their stutter and their moments of stuttering, they can begin modifying those moments and maintain a forward-flow of speech."

When we accept our stuttering, we are more likely to go forth boldly into social situations instead of hiding at home. We also tend to say even our most intimidating words—those that trip us up, which we avoided in the past.

Dropping our avoidance habits also makes us more willing to tell others that we stutter. We are more open to stuttering without feeling ashamed or embarrassed. The AIS speech therapists say this helps us to communicate effectively, even if we happen to stutter.

Like Chaya, those who reduce their avoidance often report that they are able to communicate without fear, tension, or shame, and that opens up opportunities they might not otherwise have had—like becoming speech-language pathologists who help others elevate their lives.

Origins of Avoidance Reduction Therapy

This approach was created from the 1950s through the 1970s by the late Vivien Sheehan, a speech pathologist in Los Angeles, and her late husband Joseph Sheehan, a speech pathologist and professor of psychology at UCLA.

This pioneering couple believed that stuttering was an "approach-avoidance conflict" in which the desire to speak clashed with a competing desire to hold back, because people who stuttered feared stuttering would embarrass them and make people judge them poorly.

The Sheehans believed this inner conflict not only interfered with the person's ability to communicate, but also caused inner turmoil that made daily life difficult. The couple developed a group psychotherapy approach to treating those who stuttered, encouraging clients to speak without regard to their stutters. They also encouraged them to talk about their stuttering with friends and family, which clients had never been encouraged to do previously.

The Sheehans encouraged their clients to announce their stuttering, because they believed it helped ease their fears. Eye contact was also encouraged. Their entire approach was a departure from previous stuttering treatments, which focused on slowing down and controlling speech.

The Sheehans and those who supported their approach were opposed to therapies that emphasized "fluency at any cost." They were more about encouraging clients to become more comfortable and spontaneous in their conversations, without worrying about their stuttering.

The Iceberg Analogy

The Sheehans developed the "iceberg analogy," which is often cited by speech therapists and clinicians. Dr. Sheehan noted in his 1970 book, *Stuttering: Research and Therapy*, that "stuttering is like an iceberg, with only a small part above the waterline and a much bigger part below."

They believed that our stutters are simply the most noticeable symptom, but the emotional symptoms that are less visible are really a much greater concern and need to be treated as well as our speech.

They identified seven "underwater" emotions that can have a negative impact on those of us who stutter:

1. Fear
2. Denial
3. Shame
4. Anxiety
5. Isolation
6. Guilt
7. Hopelessness

The Sheehans encouraged speech therapists and those who stutter to develop ways to reduce or eliminate the influence of each of those emotions, believing that it would improve the quality of our lives even if the stutter remains. Their approach eventually led to the development of holistic therapies, which went deeper into the emotional challenges that often accompany stuttering and make life harder for those of us who stutter.

The Sheehans told their clients that the more they tried to cover up and avoid stuttering, the more they would likely stutter. The two basic principles they encouraged clients to embrace were:

1. Stuttering doesn't hurt you.
2. Fluency doesn't do you any good.

They counseled that there is nothing to be ashamed of when you stutter, and there's nothing to be proud of when you are fluent. The Sheehans encouraged their clients to stop avoiding stuttering, and to instead speak freely without concern about it.

"See how much of the iceberg you can bring up above the surface," Joseph Sheehan wrote in his book. "When you get to the point where you're concealing nothing from your listener, you won't have much of a handicap left. You can stutter your way out of this problem if you do it courageously and openly."

Advancing, Not Avoiding

AIS client Dhruva Kathuria, now a doctoral student in the U.S., had become a master of avoidance since his childhood in India. His father also stuttered, but no one in the family ever talked about it. His father took fluency-shaping training in a city five hours away, so he'd leave for four days at a time.

Dhruva also had some fluency-shaping training, but he found it difficult to do it as well in daily conversations as he could do it in a clinical setting. While it does work for some people, most of his friends who stutter cannot use those methods effectively outside the clinic setting, he said.

Over time, Dhruva simply either avoided speaking or he spoke very slowly and tried to hide his stutter.

"I tried to speak slowly and substitute words I could say, but the authenticity of speech wasn't there. I couldn't focus on the conversation, and I substituted words so much I'd be exhausted any time I had to speak at length," he recalled in our interview.

When he came to AIS, Dhruva was surprised to find that there was not so much pressure to speak fluently, but more of an emphasis on learning to stutter without fear or anxiety. He benefitted greatly from finally beginning to break free of old avoidance habits so he could speak more comfortably with family and friends. He began online therapy with Carl Herder of AIS Atlanta in 2019 and has continued with him during his work in the PhD program in College Station, Texas.

Dhruva is a doctoral candidate at Texas A&M, specializing in the application of statistics and machine learning algorithms in agriculture. Today, this agricultural engineer aspires to become a professor, which is a big change for Dhruva. He steered clear of speaking in public for most of his life, until he learned avoidance reduction techniques from Carl.

"He went all the way up the avoidance reduction stages really quickly," the speech-language pathologist said in our interview for the book.

Dhruva developed a lot of avoidance habits including closing his eyes when he spoke. He also gestured with his arms and moved his body when trying to get through a block.

The AIS director of our Atlanta office talked with him about the underlying fears and anxieties related to his stutter, including the fact that Dhruva's mother believed he started to stutter while imitating his father. Eventually, he was able to discuss this source of tension with his family, and even to get his father to accompany him to a self-help group.

"Speaking about stuttering with them was the hardest part, because it was so sensitive in my family," Dhruva recalled. "We had never talked about it, but when we did, I learned that I had some wrong beliefs about what they thought. Once we cleared those up, I could stutter more easily."

His speech therapist also had Dhruva make five phone calls a day for a month. Later, he conducted face-to-face surveys in public, to help him face his fears of speaking. "I panicked on the first survey. I could hear my heart beating...so that was another hard thing at first," he said. "The most helpful thing was challenging my beliefs about stuttering, and those phone calls, because I had to self-advertise and do voluntary stuttering. Gradually it helped me to just force myself to be out there and do it again and again without hiding my stuttering."

Dhruva said his advice to his younger self, and to other young people who stutter, is that avoiding stuttering is not helpful in the long term. The best way to deal with those who tease you about your stuttering is to talk to them about it, instead of resenting them or hiding from them.

"Tell them that you stutter, not because you are trying to be funny or because you are not intelligent, it is because you have a speech impediment," he said. "Help them understand and they will be more sympathetic."

Dhruva learned at AIS that it is okay to stutter, and to put yourself out there because, in reality, your fears about it are usually much worse than actually speaking to people.

You shouldn't feel bad about it; in fact, many people have come around to the feeling that stuttering has made them more empathetic, compassionate, and grateful for the good in their lives. Your speech therapist will likely tell you that it may take some time to shake the avoidance habit and the behaviors that come with it, but the long-term benefits will make it worth the effort.

Stuttering for a Purpose

Avoidance reduction therapies are often paired with another treatment method called "purposeful stuttering" or "voluntary stuttering." This approach might seem counterintuitive, if not crazy, but consider that professional musicians, like those in symphony orchestras, often do something very strange when beginning a solo during a concert.

They sneak in a few bad notes. On purpose.

Musicians say this helps them feel in control, reduces anxiety, and allows them to play the rest of the solo with confidence. Speech therapists tell me that stuttering on purpose works much the same way for their clients.

Many people who stutter have learned on their own and through therapy that when they stutter on purpose and are open about their speech challenges, they tend to worry less about speaking—and as a result they struggle less with it.

Stuttering voluntarily is part of the avoidance reduction process because it helps you feel in control of your speech even as you stutter. It also puts you in a more positive frame of mind, rather than experiencing negative and self-defeating thoughts, which speech therapists call "gremlin thoughts."

Eric Dinallo is a major advocate of this method. He is the chairperson of the board of directors at AIS, a partner in the Debevoise & Plimpton law firm, and a very determined fellow. As a teenager, he decided to gain mastery over his stuttering. One of his tools was to stutter on purpose, and not just a little bit. He wrote about this in an *Atlantic* magazine story in 2019.

"One speech therapist told me that I needed to stop hiding it, and that I needed to stutter *more*. And that's exactly what I did," he wrote. "For years, I carried a counter in my pocket, like the kind used to tally people going into a stadium, and tried to voluntarily stutter 1,000 times a day."

Doing this was "exhausting," Dinallo wrote, but it forced him to shed his avoidance techniques that make speaking fluently more difficult. It also helped him move past the shame and embarrassment that is common for those who stutter.

Stuttering on purpose may sound exhausting, but as Eric notes, that is actually a small percentage of the words you typically speak every day. He tracked the number of times he stuttered on purpose by using his hand-operated counter.

"I used it even when I went on dates," he admitted in a 2017 speech for AIS.

Now, when I say Eric was determined, I mean he was *seriously* determined. In fact, he fell in a little hot water with his parents while he was home one summer from graduate school because he ran up a huge phone bill while doing his self-therapy.

"At night after everyone else went to bed, I'd set up a mirror so I could watch myself speak, and then I'd call the information operator at 411 and ask for the phone number of people with names that were very hard to pronounce. I tortured those AT&T operators," he said. "I thought it was good practice, but I had no idea that it was costing my parents a dollar a call."

Flipping the Switch

Like Eric, many clients find voluntary stuttering very helpful. They feel stuttering on purpose for their first few words helps them feel more in control of their speech. It also helps reduce their fear of stuttering involuntarily, so they see no reason to hide it.

Speech-language pathologist Carl Herder said that for some clients, even just a little practice of voluntary stuttering can be "like flipping a switch." He cautions that not everyone has the same experience, but it is not all that unusual for clients to find this method to be extremely helpful.

"We once had a client from Beirut come to our New York office and she really fought us on the concept of voluntary stuttering," Carl recalled in an interview for this book. "She said, 'Why on earth would I stutter on purpose?'"

But after she was coaxed to try this method, the client's attitude changed dramatically, as did her level of fluency and confidence, the speech-language pathologist said. "She started doing it just a little and her block disappeared, along with her fear. Once she learned to stutter on purpose instinctively, she told us, 'This is all I need to do!'"

The process of stuttering modification can often be much more complex, but my speech therapist friends tell me they witness a lot of moments in which a client will find one method, strategy, or technique that works amazingly well for them. It can be as simple as making good eye contact while stuttering and just going for it, or just forcing yourself to be more assertive, they said.

Another AIS client, Jacquelyn Jordan, an aspiring actress and screenwriter, took stuttering on purpose a step further—actually many steps further—when she decided to go out into the streets of New York City and voluntarily stutter to at least one stranger a day for one hundred days.

"I had a fear of stuttering openly…but it helps me to put it out there that I stutter," she said. "I talked to salespeople in stores and other situations, keeping it simple. My goal was just to ask a question and then I'd maintain eye contact while stuttering voluntarily."

Eye contact was important to her, because Jacquelyn tends to close her eyes when she stutters. She also challenged herself by upping the ante over her one-hundred-day challenge.

"Every twenty challenges, I'd try something else—like using a stuttering technique. Or I'd force myself to ask a follow-up question, or to say my name because I have this innate fear of saying my name," she said. "When I stutter in trying to say my name, people will say, 'What? You don't know your name?' They don't realize that I'm pausing because of the stutter, not because I don't know my own name. It's a challenge to not make that a weird moment, because at that point the stranger doesn't know you stutter."

For the most part, people were patient with her, Jacquelyn said. "Most people won't be mean to your face when you stutter on purpose to them…but if you do it on the phone, they might think it's a prank call or they lose patience, so it is easier to do in person."

Jacquelyn said that stuttering on purpose to strangers, combined with other techniques and training, helped her communicate with less fear and without obsessing over her fluency issues.

Dr. Grossman notes that the effectiveness of stuttering on purpose stems from the fact that for most people, their stutter has many layers built up over time, like the layers of an onion.

When a young child first starts to stutter, it is usually just an audible hitch. Dr. Grossman says that is the core of the "Onion of Stuttering." Other layers are added thanks to embarrassment and tension caused when someone makes fun of the child's speech at school, or the child locks up while reading aloud in class.

Once that happens, the child may avoid things—kids who tease him, talking in public, or certain words he gets stuck on, all of which adds another layer of self-doubt. The child may sense also that his parents tense up when he stutters, adding yet another layer, perhaps the fear of rejection.

The layers build and build upon each other as the child creates ways to avoid embarrassment and hurt. After so many layers, the stutter develops further because the child is trying so hard *not* to stutter, according to Dr. Grossman.

Stuttering leaves you feeling like you are out of control, so when you stutter on purpose, that fear loses some steam. Voluntary stuttering, or even just the act of letting out the stutter—with all its tension, while holding eye contact—is very therapeutic.

"By putting your stutter out there, you allow yourself to experience it without so much negative activity," Dr. Grossman says. "In real stuttering, people feel panicked and removed from communication, but with voluntary stuttering, you are right with it. You can watch for reactions in a more objective way, which is something a lot of people want to work on. They want to be able to analyze the ebb and flow of conversation, but if you are busy blocking your speech with all that drama, it is harder to do. But if you are stuttering under your own volition, it is easier to stay objective."

Proceed with Care

You should proceed with care in using this method, Carl Herder warns. He advises that you first work through your approach to stuttering on purpose with a speech therapist, because it can create problems for some people.

The concern is that someone might try to use voluntary stuttering as a method to block their involuntary stuttering, which can create more problems for them, Carl said. "But it can be helpful if someone stutters on purpose to improve their ability to move through stutters, and to prove there is no shame in stuttering," he added in our discussion for this book.

You have to be willing to put yourself out there and risk feeling uncomfortable when trying the stutter-on-purpose therapy. Some people can do it right away and even play around with it, but others need longer—occasionally a lot longer—to feel comfortable with it.

"We've had people who use this for years, keeping this method in their back pockets and pulling it out when they catch themselves feeling afraid to stutter," says Carl. "They will throw some stutters into their conversation, just to get over the fear and move on with their communication."

Speech therapists often use purposeful stuttering as a technique to desensitize their clients or audiences or to articulate a point.

"I had a client who didn't like it when I stuttered on purpose while working with her," he says. "We finally reached an agreement where she would let me stutter on purpose three times per session. Little by little, she became more accepting of it, and finally she stopped counting how many times I did it. She got more comfortable with me stuttering and with her own stuttering, but it was a slow process."

If clients are ready and willing to stutter voluntarily, it can be "extremely therapeutic," Carl Herder says.

"We do it with almost every client to help them tolerate the discomfort and to expose their stuttering to someone else."

Stuttering Rocks

Evan Sherman is another speech therapist who embraces voluntary stuttering both personally and professionally. In fact, Evan has been known to wear a wristband that reads, "Stutter like a rock star."

The Orlando-area speech therapist, who began stuttering at the age of three, remembers withdrawing from most activities in high school because of his stutter. Like many of us, his greatest nightmare was having to read aloud in class. He eventually learned to embrace the challenges by stuttering voluntarily.

"I wish I had learned voluntary stuttering early on in my life, and I wish I'd been more open about my stuttering back then," he told me in an interview for the book. "When I was sixteen or so, I started working with a therapist who took me out to stores to talk to strangers. She had me stutter voluntarily for the first time and it was the most effective thing I'd ever done."

"Voluntary stuttering was my first step towards understanding that it was okay to stutter and to be a person who stutters," he added.

Evan had avoided conversations with strangers for most of his life, but through voluntary stuttering, he learned that most did not react negatively; in fact, they listened more closely to what he said.

"If the therapist had me ask a clerk in Target where the toothbrushes were, the clerk maintained eye contact and looked at me with interest to understand what I needed," he recalled. "It was really good to see that at the time because I'd been very ashamed of my stuttering before."

As a speech therapist in private practice now, Evan considers voluntary stuttering and self-advertising to be critical tools for building confidence and reducing stress.

"A lot of stuttering occurs when you are trying not to stutter and it triggers all of these secondary avoidance characteristics," he said. "When you stutter voluntarily, your speech becomes much more forward flowing, and you feel less shame. I call it 'open stuttering.'"

He often takes his own clients to public places and has them practice self-advertising and voluntary stuttering.

"The more you can get them to talk about their stuttering in uncomfortable situations, the more comfortable they become," he said. "All of my clients have benefitted from voluntary stuttering and, honestly, it should be used in almost all therapy."

Evan even recommends that the parents of children who stutter try it themselves so they can feel firsthand what it is like to try and communicate with a stutter. "Not only will they feel what it is like to communicate that way, but they will also experience some of the anxiety and fear associated with stuttering," he said.

Evan's goal with his clients is for them to communicate what they want, when they want it, whether that be while ordering food at a restaurant or asking an employee a question in a department store.

"I want them to communicate without feelings of fear or shame or embarrassment about their stuttering," he said. "Voluntary stuttering is a key component of therapy to address these feelings and attitudes."

Stuttering with Benefits

This technique requires a lot of practice and dedication, as most need to practice using it in different situations over time to really get the full benefits. Some of the benefits include:

- Desensitizing you to stuttering so you become more confident in challenging conversations
- Finding yourself moving through stuttering and keeping the conversation flowing with less difficulty

- Easing any shame you might have over stuttering
- Helping to potentially reduce stuttering over time because of your newfound calm

Another advocate of the stuttering-on-purpose method is Peter Reitzes, who has a multi-media presence in the stuttering universe. He is a speech-language pathologist with a practice in Chapel Hill, North Carolina, as well as an author, podcaster, host, and cofounder of StutterTalk, a non-profit organization dedicated to "talking openly about stuttering."

StutterTalk is now the longest-running podcast on stuttering, with more than 675 podcasts published since 2007. It is a great resource, and Peter is very knowledgeable and helpful. He wrote a well-regarded research paper called "The Why and the How of Voluntary Stuttering" for International Stuttering Awareness Day in 2005.

I am sharing some of his thoughts from the paper with you because he makes some great points. In the paper, Peter wrote that in his view, voluntary stuttering is "the single most productive speech tool or strategy" at the disposal of adults who stutter.

He notes that stuttering on purpose when speaking to someone gets the person's stuttering out in the open, so there is no reason to hide it. The creator of StutterTalk noted that in his early twenties, he stuttered on purpose on a daily basis for more than three years. His goal was to reduce his fear of stuttering so he could say what he wanted when he wanted.

"One of my personal goals was that every time I ordered food at a restaurant or deli or asked a question in a store, I would stutter on purpose. The more I used voluntary stuttering the less I feared stuttering," he writes in "The Why and the How of Voluntary Stuttering."

With this method, you control when and how the stuttering appears, which helps stop your fear of stuttering from dominating the situation, he notes.

Another client explained that after months of stuttering on purpose, his self-image evolved from someone who hid his stutter to a person who stuttered with confidence in different situations. The result was he was able to feel like a good person even when he stuttered, not just when he was fluent.

Peter notes that some who stutter, as well as certain clinicians and family members, may question why someone would want to do more of something on purpose, when what they really want is to do less of it. There are concerns that stuttering on purpose forces clients out of their emotional comfort zones. Peter advises that most people have to practice voluntary stuttering over and over, and in a variety of situations, before they can tell if it is a helpful therapeutic tool that can be used safely.

The speech-language pathologist believes stuttering on purpose is aimed at a wide range of goals and objectives which he lists in his 2005 paper, including:

- Desensitization (reducing fear, building courage, and increasing your ability to speak in challenging communicative situations)
- Stuttering in an easy, forward-moving manner
- Increasing your ability to listen and pay attention to what others are saying
- Demonstrating that stuttering is not shameful
- Reducing moments of stuttering

Success Is the Best Revenge

Pam Mertz stutters, and is an advocate for others who stutter. She hosts a popular blog and podcast hosted on the website www.stutterrockstar.com. As someone who stuttered covertly for many years, she eventually realized "that I wasted a lot of time, and that I much prefer the authentic me," she notes on her website's "About Me" page.

Pam says her "defining moment" came when she was fired from a job that she loved and had held for more than twenty years. She knew she'd been fired because she stuttered.

"In that instant, I decided I could not live in hiding anymore and out of the closet I came," she proudly notes on her website. Now, she told me, Pam can identify two distinct phases in her life: "Fake Pam," when she was extremely covert about her stuttering, and "Real Pam," the person she was always meant to be.

It's interesting how many of us have had similar experiences. My focus and determination to overcome my stutter also motivated me to achieve success in business. So, I can identify with Pam and her story, which includes the impact that voluntary stuttering had on her life. It effectively changed her self-perception, she told me.

"They say that difficult experiences can break you or transform you. I have been transformed," she says on her website. "Since opening up about my stuttering, my world has opened up, profoundly and deeply. I feel it is my responsibility to share my journey with others whose lives have been touched by stuttering."

In a video entitled "The 411 on Voluntary Stuttering," she discusses how stuttering voluntarily can help you gain control over stuttering moments:

We often have difficulty with lack of control when we are stut-tering, which is the involuntary disruption of speech. You feel like you have no control. So, when we stutter with intent, we are in fact controlling the moment or the situation...and when we feel in control, we feel more confident and less anxious.

That is one of the reasons voluntarily stuttering is recommended as a strategy to make yourself and the listeners more comfortable. Sometimes it might be the first time a listener has heard a person who stutters, so if you are at ease, chances are the listener will relax too.

Here are a few situations when you might want to give it a try:

- Answering your cell phone
- Having dinner with family
- Ordering takeout
- Asking directions from a stranger
- Talking to your parents or spouse
- Answering a question in class or at work

My AIS friends tell me that for those of us who stutter, doing it on purpose can provide a greater sense of control. That may sound simple to people who don't have our challenges, but the range of emotions we endure often includes helplessness, shame, and embarrassment.

Stuttering voluntarily allows us to assert control, which lessens the anxiety and all of the negative emotions that can come with stuttering. My advice is to give it a try over an extended period. Give yourself time to get used to it and see how it works for you.

3

Moving Forward through Stuttering Modification

Nora O'Connor began stuttering around the age of seven. At first, she bounced off certain syllables, experienced some hesitation, and became stuck a bit more on consonants than other kids. This didn't throw her off all that much, but then the negative feedback from others began to hit home.

A waitress mocked her as she ordered a burger. One of her family members filled in a word when she got stuck. A classmate laughed when she tried to answer a question. A telephone operator hung up on her when she locked up and couldn't speak. When she met a cute boy in junior high, she couldn't get her name out to introduce herself.

Everyone who stutters has similar stories of those awful experiences that made us realize we were "different" and easily teased and mocked.

For Nora, and so many others, that initial realization gave rise to fears and insecurities that seemed to snowball into a form of paralysis, she noted in a 2002 paper she wrote on self-image issues.

"Every decision, every move, every breath revolved around my disfluencies," Nora recalled.

Her frustration also reflected the fact that the only others she knew who stuttered were boys. She felt unfairly burdened and alone. She tried therapy a couple times during her school years without success.

Before she sought treatment for her stuttering again as an adult, Nora silenced herself and withdrew from others. She had no goals for her life, except to "stay quiet, hidden, and wither away."

Today, she is a clinical social worker and therapist who counsels young people and adults who stutter, along with many other clients in Los Angeles. She has been featured in two documentaries on stuttering, *Spit It Out* and *Right Here, Right Now*.

Before she became a nationally known advocate for those who stutter, Nora was just like many young people with this challenge. She felt that her low self-esteem and lack of coping skills were normal for someone who stuttered and that little was expected of her or from her.

"I wasn't up to the task of squaring off against that monster called stuttering. Stuttering was simply too powerful. It sapped every ounce of my strength. In my frustration, exhaustion, and isolation, I used to think...it's not supposed to be this way. I'm *too good* to be silenced like this! I have too much to say. Too much to do. Too much to contribute, to just stand silently on the sidelines of life."

Every time she tried to rise above those negative feelings and insecurities, it seemed something slapped her down and she'd come away "more terrified than before, more reluctant to ever try again."

Sadly, Nora summed up her life like this: "I wasn't a girl living with stuttering. I was a girl *dying* with stuttering."

Eventually, she would find the help she desperately needed from friends, family, other women with stutters, a speech therapist, and a psychotherapist. They helped her get to the root of her insecurities and fear, which was her inner war with stuttering.

One of the several techniques that Nora benefitted from in her speech therapy was stuttering modification, which involves physical retraining that teaches you to "catch" a moment of stuttering and then reduce the tension enough that you can keep moving forward in your speech.

Some call this "easy stuttering" because it allows you to begin speaking and move more smoothly through stuttering moments. A speech therapist will have you practice a word, such as "soda," by having you prolong the "s" and then gently initiate the "o" vowel to keep you progressing through the word.

This form of more gentle stuttering helps you lay the groundwork for transforming the hitches in your speech into a smoother flow that gives you more space to be comfortable and thoughtful, and less overwhelmed and panicky. The goal is to help you feel more in control of your speech so you feel less tension, and to help increase your awareness of moments when you stutter and how you can manage them with greater confidence.

The benefits of this strategy include:

- Less tension
- A greater sense of awareness and control
- A more relaxed speech flow
- Less struggling with speech
- A more positive attitude about communicating

- A feeling of acceptance while being more open and expressive
- The ability to take control

The AIS approach with stuttering modification therapy does not target fluency, but instead works to change how we stutter by teaching us three points at which you can modify your stuttering, either before, during, or after the block in your speech.

The AIS Approach

Preparatory Set

This is a modification you can do *before* you hit a block. So, as you approach a word you think you might block on, you use a technique often called "easing out" or "bouncing," or "easy bouncing." *(Carl Herder explains that many speech therapists avoid assigning terms to techniques because sometimes clients get too focused on the name or jargon. Even so, there are many avid proponents of this strategy and many who've found it very helpful in their daily lives, often in combination with other therapeutic approaches.)*

In this type of voluntary stuttering, you slow down repetitions in a relaxed way to move your speech forward, lessening your tendency to avoid stuttering and avoiding your negative reactions to it. The idea is to move through the block by reducing the physical tension—but you don't have to do it perfectly. Sometimes it's not always easy to reduce all of the tension, which is natural. Even reducing just some of the tension can be very helpful, since this technique encourages you to be more comfortable with moments of stuttering.

Pullouts

This is the modification you can use *during* a stutter block. It involves altering a stutter as it occurs, replacing a hard stutter with an easy stutter to help ease tension as we complete the word. This is accomplished when you notice a stutter occurring and respond by slowing down, stretching, and smoothing out the transition between sounds as you finish the word.

Sometimes clients will do a natural pullout as they get better at monitoring their physical tension and secondary behaviors, such as closing their eyes or avoiding eye contacts. Speech therapists recommend modifying in the moment to come out of the stutter in a more relaxed way.

Cancellations

This modification is used *after* you stutter on a word. You immediately repeat the word you've stuttered on, but with greater ease and a more "fluent" stutter. For example: "*M-M-M-Message…message.*" The idea is to improve the flow of your speech and gain more confidence as you go.

Learning Not to Fight with Your Stutter

In Nora O'Connor's case, stuttering modification alone did not "cure" all of her communication challenges, nor did it alleviate all of her fears and insecurities. Yet, when combined with other methods—developed over years of therapy and counseling— Nora has learned to live on her own terms, while building an accomplished and remarkable life. As Nora notes in her writings and interviews, she still deals with her root problem of stuttering every day, as well as the negative thoughts and feelings associated with it.

"Today, my stuttering and who I am are no longer two separate entities. Now they are one in the same, and usually in harmony with each other. True, there are times when the old negative thinking rears its ugly head, and my thoughts threaten again to overpower me," she explains in her paper "Self-Image Issues."

"But I no longer fight that voice; I hear what it has to say and then I let it go. It's been a long, challenging quest from where I was to where I am today; and now, at last, when I look in the mirror, I am proud of the self-image I have created as a woman living with stuttering."

Stuttering Modification vs. Fluency Shaping

There are two primary approaches to direct speech therapy. One is stuttering modification, sometimes called "easy stuttering," which was explored above.

The other approach is fluency shaping, also known as speech restructuring. This method was developed by the famed clinical psychologist Dr. Ronald Webster, the founder of Hollins Communications Research Institute in Roanoke, Virginia.

With stuttering modification, the primary focus is on working with the stutter to make it flow more quickly, with less tension so the client is more comfortable. The main goal with fluency shaping, on the other hand, is to stop stuttering as much as possible so the client's speech is fluent and fast.

While it seems to make more sense to try and eliminate stuttering altogether, many believe that implementing fluency shaping to stop stuttering entirely is much more difficult to master than stuttering modification, which allows for stuttering without the anxiety that often accompanies it.

Stuttering modification was originally developed in the 1930s by Charles Van Riper, a speech-learning pathologist who stuttered. The speech therapists at AIS use it to help clients physically change their stuttering while working on avoidance, feelings, and attitudes.

In a nutshell, the goal of fluency shaping is to help you achieve maximum fluency without stuttering. The goal of stuttering modification, in contrast, is to change moments of stuttering so that the client is more relaxed, less concerned about how others react, and feels more in control and free to speak without being perfectly fluent.

There are those in the stuttering community who strongly favor one over the other, and some who think both have their benefits and their downsides. There are therapeutic programs that offer training in both, so clients have different options and tools. My goal is just to give you a good understanding of both, and then let you and your speech therapist decide what's best for you.

Reducing the Struggle

You may never completely eliminate your stutter, but stuttering modification alleviates the struggle, which is often the biggest burden of all.

"We want people to understand that this may not go away but they don't have to struggle with it and hate it all their lives," Carl Herder of AIS told me. "In fact, many people develop an appreciation for their stutter because there are so many life lessons to be learned from the experience."

Carl worked with a client named Rose, who practiced pull-outs during stuttering modification training. In a video with Carl on the AIS website, Rose explained, "You actually get a chance to notice how much force you have when you are blocking and when you use [the stuttering modification], it feels so different and your blocks are not so severe."

Rose said she envisioned reducing the tension on a block, dialing it down mentally from nine to nothing, and it helped her make smoother transitions in her speaking…even more than she'd expected.

"It actually helps a lot," she said. "When I first started, most of my stuttering was blocking and it was very tiring and very debilitating, almost, because you are trying to force everything out."

The stuttering modification methods helped Rose create a "clean stutter," that was not as difficult as her previous stutter because she no longer fell into using avoidance habits that made her stutter worse.

Bouncing to Better Communication

Jai Prakash "J.P." Sunda felt his stutter was so bad that he'd never get an IT job after graduating from college in his native India. He was surprised, then, when he did get an offer, but he was also quite nervous.

J.P. realized that, for the first time, he'd be on a team working in close quarters. There would be "no escape" from speaking to others, he said in a StutterTalk interview with Peter Reitzes.

His fear of stuttering initially affected his job performance so much that he feared his boss might fire him. J.P. went to a speech therapist, and for the first time in his life, someone told him that "it was okay to stutter."

This encouraged him, easing some of the fears he felt about communicating with others. But what really made the difference was learning the stuttering modification technique known as "bouncing," which is a form of stuttering on purpose.

At first, he felt ashamed to use this technique—from a young age, he'd been taught to focus on achieving fluency. But eventually, J.P. found the courage to begin stuttering voluntarily.

In group therapy with others who stuttered, he learned to use pullouts as well as bouncing—repeating the first syllable of a word on purpose a few times to move through a block.

"I started realizing if these guys are doing it and sound so comfortable with their stammers, maybe even I can try it," he told Reitzes, who you may remember is a speech-language pathologist and the founder of StutterTalk.

Over time, J.P. began to feel more in control and less fearful of speaking to others. Eventually, he even created a local support group, which led to his becoming the coordinator of a national group called the Indian Stammering Association.

His journey from being fearful of the most routine communications to leading a national organization for those who stutter is inspiring for those of us who've dealt with the same fears and challenges.

"I was always anxious and afraid. I became a very timid person and it was very hard to live that way," he said in the podcast. "If I had a meeting after lunch, it would be hard to eat the lunch. Then, when you are ordering lunch, that was stressful itself. You'd think, 'What do I want to eat, and will I be able to say it?'"

J.P. said that after learning stuttering modification, he would stammer on purpose while ordering his meal. This method calmed him, allowing him to enjoy his meal and the rest of his workday.

Over time, he became willing to stutter in public and to talk about stuttering openly.

He found stuttering modification to be liberating to the point that this once timid and reclusive young man even began speaking to schoolchildren, teachers, and principals as an advocate and source of inspiration for those who stutter. Those meetings, in turn, gave him even more confidence and led to less stuttering.

"My increase in fluency is largely due to my willingness to stammer openly and talk about my stuttering openly," he said. "I unintentionally became so open about my stutter by talking about it at so many schools with teachers and children and bouncing a lot, there was an increase in fluency."

J.P.'s old fears occaisionally pop up now and then, especially when someone reacts to his stuttering in a strange way. But even when that happens, J.P. reaches into his stuttering modification toolbox and uses the tools he has mastered.

"Once in a while—when I get those bad experiences or weird looks—it helps me more. It helps me also to be at peace and learn how to handle such reactions, so when they happen, I'm glad they do," he said.

In June of 2020, J.P. and his wife immigrated to Canada and began a new life there together. He was given a big send-off by his many friends and fans at the Indian Stammering Association (stammer.in) and he plans on continuing to post updates on their website and Facebook pages. In an email to me, he also offered these words of encouragement for all of those who stutter:

When we allow ourselves to be as we are, then the "improvement" happens naturally. Just be present in the moment and allow whatever the moment presents to happen naturally, whether it is stammering or anything else. That is the foundation. And yes, the whole journey may [...] sound linear, yet, it is anything but that. It is mostly one step forward and one step backward.

4

Hello, I Stutter,
Get Over It, I Did!

College students can be a tough audience. Graduate students are even more challenging. They tend to be very serious about learning what they need to know so they can get out into the world, apply it, and start a career.

I know this because for fourteen years, I was an adjunct professor at the Fordham University Gabelli School of Business. I also founded the Fordham Leadership Forum there, which provides MBA students with lectures by top business leaders.

You may have noticed by now that for a guy with a lifelong stutter, I didn't exactly avoid speaking in public. That doesn't mean it was easy. Holding their attention was often a struggle.

I eventually figured out that the best approach was to be very direct. Every day, the first words out of my mouth to my twenty-five or so grad students was: "I have a speech impediment. I stutter, and sometimes I will be disfluent."

I let them know that I might stutter occasionally. When I told them up front, I felt calmer, and because they knew a hitch or two might be coming, they were more comfortable, too.

This method is known by a variety of names in the stuttering community—self-advertising, announcing, and disclosure are just a few I've heard used. To those who don't stutter, this method might sound very simple and sensible. Sure, why not just tell everyone off the bat that you stutter? Makes sense!

But those of us who do stutter usually carry so much baggage, so many fears and anxieties and dreads, that this method isn't quite as easy as it may sound to those who naturally experience fluent speech.

Believe me, someone who stutters has to work long and hard to get to the point where they can discuss their stutter in front of a group of strangers, or even people they may know well. Yet, my speech therapist and speech pathologist friends tell me that self-advertising has helped many of their clients over the years, often in combination with other therapies.

Former AIS client Michael Taub shared a story on the AIS blog about his experiences in self-advertising his stutter when he became a student teacher in a middle school. He prefaced his story by noting that "sometimes when I find myself speaking almost fluently for a good amount of time, I think, 'Look at how far I've come.' What usually happens then is that I start getting hung up on not stuttering…and I start silent blocking more."

Michael said that this is a cycle he falls into: stuttering, managed fluency paired with bouts of spontaneous fluency and bursts of confidence, and then moments of uncertainty.

Many of us who stutter experience the same or similar cycles with our stuttering challenges. Michael says self-advertising is the tool that helps him the most. "Without advertising, I don't know how I would've dealt with one of my bigger more recent challenges."

Here is Michael's story, as told in the AIS blog:

I began my middle school student teaching placement a month ago as part of the process to become a state-certified social studies teacher. This wasn't going to be my first time in front of a classroom. I taught English for a couple of years in Ecuador, and this past fall semester I student taught 11th graders in a South Bronx high school. However, because this was going to be my first attempt at teaching young kids, I felt like the stakes were high.

I wanted to show myself that I had a newfound confidence that I lacked in 1998 as a middle school student. I wanted to show myself that adult me could stutter without fear and shame. I wanted to show the middle school students that I was a confident teacher.

When I was in middle school, I was always trying to blend in with the rest of the kids. Before I started getting serious about dealing with my stuttering, the last thing I wanted to do was draw attention to what I used to consider a weakness.

So now, there I was—standing in front of 27 twelve and thirteen-year-olds, part of me feeling like I was in eighth grade again, as if I was about to deliver an oral report that I had been dreading for days. I could hear my cooperating teacher's voice and suddenly I was half-dreaming. "Mr. Taub will be with us through the spring. Mr. Taub, is there anything you'd like to say to the class...?"

Everything seemed surreal. I reminded myself of some of the experiences from the past decade that separated adult me from teenage me... "I'm looking forward to working with you guys. Oh and, one more thing. I w-w-w-want to let you know that I stutter, which means that sometimes I repeat my words or syllables or speak slowly. I'm fine with it, so if you ever have questions about it or if you need me to repeat myself, just ask."

Some kids looked surprised. Some didn't. I chose not to worry either way.

At the end of the third class on that first day, a co-teacher in one of our integrated "mainstream" and special education classes said to me, "You know, this is really going to be great for John."

She pointed to a student putting a notebook into his backpack, pushing his chair back under the table. "John stutters, and he's going to enjoy having you in the classroom." And I remembered again why I'm proud to be a person who stutters.

Being Up Front

Michael Taub, who is now in the healthcare field, is just one of many who have learned how the seemingly simple act of telling people that they stutter can have a powerful impact on their lives.

When former AIS client George Daquila interviewed for his dream job as a software programmer for Goldman Sachs in New York City, he did not try to hide his stutter.

In fact, George, who is now a vice president at Goldman Sachs, put it right out there first thing, with each and every step of the interview process, he wrote in a 2016 article in *Letting Go*, an online newsletter for westutter.org (a website of the National Stuttering Association).

"I told everyone up front, because I've found that it relaxes me and relaxes the person I'm talking to. I explain how stuttering used to hold me back, but through a lot of hard work, I came out stronger," he said in the article. "That led to some in-depth conversations with the managers interviewing me, and I could tell it impressed them."

As discussed previously, this method has a few names, such as self-disclosure. It works in much the same way as stuttering on purpose, because it helps reduce the stress and fear that often accompany stuttering.

"Sometimes I will bring up the topic of stuttering and it is always a positive experience. People will ask questions, which gives me a deeper connection with that person. It exposes me and shows that I can be open, which always has a positive effect on the conversation or relationship," he explains.

The workplace presents special challenges to those of us who stutter. George Daquila advocates disclosing your stuttering as the best way to navigate those challenges. Here are four tips he has offered on the AIS website:

1. Be willing to disclose your stuttering. Willingness is step one. George says to ask yourself: "Am I willing to disclose that I stutter?" If the answer is yes, great! Check in with the following three basic steps and you're ready to go. If the answer is no, that's okay too. You might want to then consider exploring with a good friend, trusted mentor, or speech therapist what to do next in order to get ready for that first step.

2. Start with the people you are most comfortable with; then, as you get comfortable, expand beyond your inner circle— for example, friends at work—to build a support network and to gain confidence.

3. Challenge yourself to advertise your stutter in safe but bold and fun ways. You can do this by voluntarily stuttering, disclosing more, or creating mock interviews for people who stutter in your workplace (like George does). Pushing your comfort zone will keep you in good "stuttering shape." As George says, "the work is never done," so find ways that you can challenge yourself that are safe, fun, and effective.

4. Think of your stutter as an asset that makes you stronger, more resilient, and a more valuable person to have around.

Powering Up

Although George has struggled with feelings of shame and fear as a child and even into adulthood, he has succeeded in his career by approaching his work with this attitude of self-confidence. As a software programmer, he spends his days speaking to co-workers, traders, business partners, and portfolio managers. He needs to interact with them and collaborate with his team members to create the software they need.

Like most of us, George had to work hard and overcome a lot of emotional baggage to get to that point. He dreaded speech therapy in grade school because the emphasis was on perfecting speech fluency, and that approach only left him feeling shamed and embarrassed.

"The therapist was an absolutely wonderful person," he said in the *Letting Go* article. "But this didn't work for me at all."

Later, his parents found a speech therapist who worked with George to accept his speaking challenges. For the first time, he used the term "stuttering" during speech therapy, but, he said, he still had a lot of shame that made him hide.

Most of us have our ups and downs with stuttering. We can go for long periods when it doesn't bother us, and then all of a sudden, something happens to trigger the negative emotions that can accompany a lack of fluency. George stopped therapy in college because he was doing so well, but then he had a "slow degrading of [his] confidence and speech." He struggled in graduate school, so he went to a counselor for psychotherapy, which he described as "an amazing experience." George also decided to videotape himself in different speaking situations as self-therapy.

This proved to be a painful experience, so he began speech therapy again, working more on self-acceptance as well as fluency. He regained his confidence to the point that he would bring up his stuttering in social conversations. Self-advertising worked well for him and gave him the self-assurance to move out of academia and into the fast-paced and highly collaborative world of high-finance IT.

While he doesn't shy away from acknowledging that those who stutter face difficult challenges, George believes that being open about it puts him on the road to less stress and anxiety. "You need to be ruthless with yourself and face it head on," he said in the *Letting Go* article. "I used to think that I was weak because I stuttered, but it has made me much stronger."

Putting It Out There

Like George and me, speech-language pathologist Carl Herder is another big fan of being up front and open about stuttering.

"It is always something we have encouraged and trained people to do because this method can make a big difference," Carl said. "We want people to be more authentically themselves. Those who stutter can get caught up and bogged down in what others might think of them or how they might react, but sharing an acknowledgment about stuttering up front often frees them up to get back to the business of communicating openly and freely."

Just a few years ago, speech therapists often suggested that those who stutter make their disclosures or self-advertise in ways that were subtle and perhaps even a little apologetic.

"We had them say things like 'I stutter, so please be patient and bear with me, the words will come out eventually.' It wasn't an explicit apology, but it had an apologetic feel to it," he said. "With that approach, you were kind of asking the listener to do something extra and pay more attention while demonstrating patience."

The latest approach to disclosure is more assertive in tone, Carl explained.

For example, on a telephone call with someone you haven't met, the person who stutters might say up front, "Hey, just so you know, I stutter, so you might notice a delay in my speech. It isn't a bad phone connection; I'm just having a block in my speech. I promise the words will come out eventually."

Many find that trying to suppress stuttering at work can be wearing, stressful, and hurt your effectiveness. So, by putting your stutter out there, you will likely find you have more mental energy to devote to doing your job.

Mark O'Malia, a speech therapist in the AIS New York City office, has noted that many of his clients have embraced stuttering disclosure, especially in the workplace, as a way to normalize it.

Mark knows lawyers and medical professionals who use self-advertising to educate their co-workers, clients, and patients. Announcing your stutter also helps to counter any overt or subtle forms of discrimination in those hyper-competitive fields. Many who stutter agree with Mark that telling people up front about your stutter can be very beneficial, because the self-disclosure tends to break down walls and ease discomfort in both parties, helping to establish an immediate connection.

Often, the more open someone is about stuttering, the higher that person's self-esteem becomes, according to the experiences of AIS therapists. Opening up a conversation by saying that you stutter seems to work best if you are direct, confident, and unapologetic. Humor is always a good approach, too: "Hi, nice to meet you. I stutter, so if some words aren't rolling off my tongue, just give me a minute. I'll get them to you before the end of the day…usually!"

Self-disclosing is very helpful, especially to people who tend to fret about what other people might be thinking when they stutter. Just getting it out there eliminates that concern right away, right? Talking openly about your stuttering also shows that you accept yourself as a fallible human being, perfectly imperfect, just like everyone else on the planet.

Now, when I recommend this method, some people say, "What should I call it?"

Well, that's a simple one. Call it *stuttering*! Unless you live in England, where they call it *stammering*.

The bottom line is, stuttering isn't contagious or lethal, so you shouldn't feel the need to apologize. It isn't your fault, and don't dwell on it. Tell 'em what it is and move on, because you have interesting things to say!

The actor Harvey Keitel often talks openly about his stuttering in interviews and speeches. In a 1995 *Washington Post* interview, he described his stutter as "something that occurs as the result of something else.… It's sort of a road to your identity, it's a clue about something, it's a clue about disturbance."

Mark O'Malia used self-disclosure to help overcome his own fears of stuttering, and now he teaches it to his clients. "After I learned to just tell people I stuttered, life opened up to me. I didn't have perfect fluency, but I believed I could handle any speaking situation thrown my way, and I could pursue my passions in life," he said.

Mark and other speech therapists caution that being a person who stutters can be tough, but trying to hide it—and suppress the negative feelings that can arise—will only make the challenges greater. Most people discover that the more they talk openly about stuttering, the less of an issue it seems.

The Subway Challenge

As a New Yorker, I have spent many hours riding the subway. It has never occurred to me to announce to my fellow passengers that I have a stutter, but that is exactly what the speech therapists at AIS have done with some clients.

They call this the "Subway Challenge."

Be aware that this exercise is not a mandatory part of the intensive program at AIS. It is purely voluntary, but many clients embrace this challenge and go for it. I personally haven't ever wanted to do the Subway Challenge, but if others want to do it, that is their choice. It takes some guts. New Yorkers, after all, are known as the world's toughest audience.

The Subway Challenge originated years ago with an AIS client named Ben, who had a severe stutter. He enrolled in the intensive therapy program with great enthusiasm, and had no fear when it came to announcing his stutter while making telephone calls or talking to strangers in shops and parks.

Ben found the concept of public disclosure to be very therapeutic and liberating. One day while riding the subway, he was inspired to take it to another level. He stood up and declared to his fellow passengers that he had a stutter.

This was not part of the AIS program. He did it entirely on his own. The people on the subway responded well, so he began doing it nearly every trip he took. Ben shared this experience with others who stuttered and soon they were doing it too.

AIS client Jacquelyn Joyce was one of the few people to find the Subway Challenge problematic, but her reasons had more to do with a general discomfort with riding the subway than with how people responded to her. A native of Los Angeles, Jacquelyn earned a master's degree in theater in New York City, and along the way she developed the feeling that the subway was for transportation, not communication.

"Taking the subway is scary enough for regular people, so putting the added pressure of self-advertising my stutter on the subway was not fun for me, even though the reception from other riders was mostly congratulatory," she said.

"Some people clapped when I stood up and said I stutter, but it didn't feel authentic to me. I mean, it was cool in the moment, but I wouldn't do it again. New York City is so fast paced. When I lived there, I was taking the subway all the time, and the last thing I wanted while riding it was for other people to talk to me.

"I just wanted to get to my final destination. So, I didn't want anyone imposing on my time on the subway and that was a consideration for me during the Subway Challenge. I wasn't comfortable imposing on them."

Jacquelyn said self-advertising does work for her in other settings. She uses it often, especially now that she is busy doing podcasts and interviews. Now back in Los Angeles, where she returned to care for a mother with dementia, she has focused on screenwriting. She created an inspirational short film series that runs on YouTube and has earned some media attention.

"Whenever I do an interview or a podcast, I start out by saying, 'I just want you to know I have a stutter,' and I've found that when I do that, the pressure to be fluent no longer weighs on me."

5

Taking Control through Fluency Shaping Therapy

Co-anchoring a network news show seems like an unlikely job for someone who spent most of his life living in fear of stuttering publicly. Yet, John Stossel is a familiar face and name to viewers who've seen him on *Good Morning America, 20/20,* and Fox Business News during his television career of more than forty years.

For most people, it's hard to imagine that Stossel was once yanked off the air as a young reporter because of his stutter. He was so traumatized by that incident that during his six years as co-anchor of ABC's *20/20* news program with Barbara Walters, he did all of his reports on videotapes, which could be edited if he stuttered.

To alleviate his stutter, John tried acupuncture, hypnosis, transcendental meditation, and intense therapy programs, without a great deal of success. He eventually did much better by relentlessly practicing fluency shaping therapy techniques, which include breathing in before talking and speaking softly and slowly.

As mentioned in Chapter 3, Dr. Ron Webster developed this method of "easy stuttering" promoted by the HCRI. John Stossel and I are among many others who have benefitted tremendously from the programs at Hollins. Dr. Webster's national stuttering research center has been of immense help to me over the years, since I first went through a three-week program about forty years ago.

Before I went to Hollins, I had struggled with a stutter all of my life. I grew up in an Orthodox Jewish home in Brooklyn. Hebrew school was especially difficult for me because of my stutter. I knew the answers, but when I couldn't get them out quickly enough, the rabbi spanked me. My concerned mother scraped together what she could and sent me to the National Hospital for Speech Disorders, but nothing they offered really worked for me. Back then, they mostly tried to teach you how to live with your stutter.

Well into my twenties, I tried every program known to man to stop stuttering, but still struggled. Ironically, I became a speechwriter for my commanding officer while serving in the U.S. Army. The general was a former attaché for President John F. Kennedy, and when I returned to civilian life, I was hired as a speechwriter for his brother Robert Kennedy while he was running for the U.S. Senate. Later, I was recruited to work for a leading company, Lederle Laboratories (now Pfizer), in the pharmaceutical industry. I was determined not to let my stuttering hold me back in my career. Coming up in corporate life and feeling nervous about my speech, I told myself, "You're not going to get the job if you can't get your name out."

Many of those who stutter go into IT or engineering, where they don't have to talk a lot. Very few are crazy like me and go into marketing and public relations.

I was already in my thirties when I enrolled in the speech fluency program at Hollins, shortly after it opened. I went to their satellite campus in New Paltz, New York, on weekends, and basically learned to speak all over again. I then did the annual three-day workshops every summer for fifteen years. This method helped smooth out my speech and build my confidence. I still use many of the techniques and training methods I learned there to help my level of fluency.

Over time, I went from having a moderate stutter to a mild one. I was so grateful that a friend and I set up a scholarship, and each year we send three young people to the institute. (A lot of them stay in touch, writing me letters. I ask them to call instead, so I can hear how they sound.)

Most who stutter will take jobs where they can hide their stutter, but I had wanted to be a CEO since I was a kid. I always felt I wasn't going to let this impediment stand in my way.

Muscling Through

Fluency shaping therapy, along with a lot of hard work and perseverance, helped me achieve my dreams. Dr. Webster and his research team have developed a comprehensive behavioral stuttering therapy. Their research has shown that stuttering is a physically based phenomenon with genetic origins.

Their program is designed to teach those who stutter how to replace faulty speech muscle movements that cause stuttering with new muscle behaviors that generate fluent speech. They have treated more than 6,500 clients from fifty countries and all walks of life.

I believe Dr. Webster, now in his seventies, is a brilliant man. He has been working for years with the National Institutes of Health to look into the genetic origins of stuttering. That makes sense to me, because I had an uncle who stuttered, and many others who stutter have relatives with the same challenge. Dr. Webster said his research has found that about half of those who stutter have family members who share that challenge.

Researchers from the NIH believe gene variations may explain why that is true. Their findings add to evidence that stuttering is rooted in the complex interaction of genetics, brain wiring, and muscles that control speech. "At this point, the research team has identified four mutant genes identified with stuttering in about 20 percent of cases," Dr. Webster told me recently. "We are looking into doing a genetic analysis on people before they come to therapy with the idea that we may be able to make the program more powerful for people who have the gene or genes."

The Complex Mechanics of Speaking

Dr. Webster noted that there are forty-four basic sounds in the American English language, but over ten thousand different syllables that are very distinctive and different across families of sound, with a vast complexity of how sounds interact with each other that has to be taken into account.

"It is important to know how it is complex and what to do about those complexities," he explained in our interview for the book. "Speech sounds do not string together like beads on a chain when we talk. They don't follow like letters appearing on a screen typed on a keyboard. The same sound at the beginning of a word is changed in its physical form by the sounds that come afterwards, and this is where the complexities come in."

Most people are not conscious of the physical mechanics of speaking, such as their breathing, tone of voice, and the movements of their lips, tongues, and jaws. Fluency shaping therapy trains those who stutter how to slow down their speech and consciously control those mechanics.

The training begins with you speaking almost in a monotone, almost like a robot, and then gradually advancing to more normal-sounding speech. You learn how to control your breathing during conversations, how to adjust your articulation with your lips, jaw, and tongue, to control the tension in your voice, to stretch out vowels and consonants, and to slow the rate of your speaking.

Once you master these techniques, which can take a long time and require constant practice, you can gradually increase the speed and vary the tones in your speaking. Again, this takes a great deal of determination and hard work. I still have to work at it, and my fluency varies, but as Dr. Webster noted in our interview, "Sander has been very consistent in trying to stick with the target behavior that generates fluency. He has a great attitude and may be a little variable in his performance, but then, we are all variable in how we perform, whether it is in speaking, sports performance, or playing music."

Of course, the training at Hollins has evolved over the years since I first attended classes. Dr. Webster says their modern approach is "much more cognizant of the details of what your speech muscles are doing and what they must be trained to do." The number of target behaviors has probably doubled from when I began my speech therapy at Hollins, according to the founder. In fact, Dr. Webster told me recently:

Instructions have been refined and tested, and if we give you an instruction, we know that hundreds of people have responded well to it. All of our programs have been refined and polished. The most important technical development is we have improved our ability to measure what your speech muscles are doing by analyzing the sounds coming out of your mouth. We are much better and more precise with our feedback, and the quantification has gotten better.

There Is an App for That, but Practice Is Still Essential

Dr. Webster recently told me that they have created an HCRI app for the iPhone that is virtually a "clinician in your pocket." Available only to our clients, this app evaluates, scores, and provides immediate feedback on speech skills taught during HCRI therapy.

"You can open it up and talk to the iPhone to monitor the quality of your speech. It's a pretty clever tool and holds you to certain performance standards," he said.

Even with all the advances, the Hollins fluency shaping therapy requires ten to twelve hours a week of practice.

"Speech is complex, and therapy needs to take that into account, otherwise people will fail," he said. "We've made almost all the mistakes that can be made to get to where we are now with our work. We don't want to be dogmatic, but we can tell you what we have done that has been successful and what has not been successful."

The Hollins approach differs from many others in that Dr. Webster's training focuses more on voice control and physically controlling speech, rather than the emotional aspects of stuttering.

Dr. Webster believes focusing on treating the emotions around stuttering amounts to "attaching the cart to the wrong end of the horse." The Hollins founder believes the emotional aspects and reactive aspects of stuttering come from the fact that speech muscles are breaking down and the patterns of movement are being inhibited and blocked. These struggles, in turn, trigger emotional reactions—like frustration and embarrassment for those who stutter. On his methodical approach, Dr. Webster explained to us:

> *If we clear out blockages, your emotions change rather quickly and substantially, because you know directly what you can do to generate fluent speech. Our recommendation is that you look carefully at the physical side of what is happening when you stutter, and then seek therapy that deals directly with the misbehavior of speech muscles in a comprehensive and systematic way. If you try to make stuttering simpler than it really is, you will probably have to live with it because it is not going to get better.*

Grateful Grads

John Stossel and I have been very public in expressing our gratitude to the team at Hollins, and Dr. Webster notes that there are many other success stories out there. One such client was a young medical school applicant who couldn't get through his first interview, but after fluency training at Hollins, he went on to become a successful physician.

Dr. Webster also offered the story of a major in the military who stuttered, and had decided he would retire if he failed one more evaluation for a promotion in rank. "He went through our program, did a great job, and got his promotion to lieutenant colonel, who briefed generals in the Pentagon," the proud founder said.

Dr. Webster noted that Hollins alumni have included members of royal families in other nations, as well as the late Annie Glenn, wife of the late astronaut and U.S. Senator John Glenn.

While her husband was celebrated as a hero for his exploits in space, Mrs. Glenn struggled with a stutter so severe that she could only say about 15 percent of what she wanted to express. She tried several different speech therapy programs, but felt most of them made her feel better, not speak better.

Mrs. Glenn often said that she became "an expert at being seen and not heard" when accompanying her husband during his career as an astronaut and politician. She often resorted to writing things out for salesclerks, taxi drivers, and restaurant staff when her husband or other family and friends weren't around.

Finally, at the age of fifty-three, Mrs. Glenn took the intensive program at Hollins in 1973 as part of their first big group of clients. Two weeks into the program, she found herself speaking at a normal rate and confidently making phone calls for the first time in her life.

Eventually, Annie Glenn became a polished public speaker who moved audiences to tears with her story. She returned to Hollins a couple times to try out new therapies over the years. As she noted in a 1980 *People* magazine interview, and in many other press interviews and speeches, "I used to be just a good listener; now I'm a chatterbox."

Mrs. Glenn became a spokesperson for national organizations for those who stutter, and served as an inspiration for many people faced with the same challenges. Dr. Webster told me that her greatest pride was reading to her grandchildren, something she couldn't do for her own children when they were growing up.

Mrs. Glenn always made a point to say that fluency shaping may not work for everyone, but it certainly worked for her. Annie was a wonderful friend to me.

Over the years, fluency shaping has helped thousands of people, including Annie Glenn, John Stossel, and me. Our speech isn't always perfect, but as John has noted, we no longer have the fear and anxiety that can aggravate the problems for those who stutter. As John told the Stuttering Foundation in a speech, "Fear of stuttering can easily become worse than the stuttering itself. The idea that I'm on television and making speeches is still a shock to me sometimes."

The Pros and Cons of Fluency Shaping

Today, many therapy programs use fluency shaping in combination with other methods to serve each individual's special needs and challenges. AIS, which I also support by providing scholarships and serving on the board, has moved away from emphasizing fluency shaping therapies in more recent years.

Their speech therapists and pathologists tend to use fluency shaping mostly with clients who request it, or have issues with speech rates or managing their speech.

"We could use fluency shaping just to help clients start speaking more gently, or working on a more measured rate of speech by elongating syllables or prolonging them to help them speak in an easier and more relaxed manner," said Carl Herder, the AIS speech-language pathologist in Atlanta, in our interview.

In their fluency shaping therapy, the AIS approach focuses on the physical sensation of vocal fold/cord vibration and diaphragmatic breathing to help clients first slow down their speech and then ease into a more natural rate.

Benefits of Fluency Shaping Therapy

Carl Herder noted the benefits of the fluency shaping therapy include:

1. Perfecting fluency in certain situations. Most clients can achieve perfect fluency in the clinical setting, which helps them feel more confident, especially if they can continue to do that in real-life situations outside the clinic for extended periods.

2. Giving clients something tangible to work on. This therapy provides clients and their loved ones with the feeling that they are taking positive steps to address fluency issues. It helps reduce feelings of helplessness and frustration.

3. Increasing the client's mindfulness about speech mechanisms.

4. Offering relaxation, almost like meditation, because of the long vocalization exercises.

5. Producing more feelings of control in their speech, which is empowering.

6. Boosting confidence!

7. Teaching that by working hard and focusing, they can produce a positive difference in their lives.

Drawbacks of Fluency Shaping Therapy

The AIS speech pathologists and therapists also shared some of the drawbacks they see in this form of therapy. They note that the drawbacks are complex because of the paradox involved.

AIS Director Dr. Heather Grossman explained:

> *In my opinion, while working on fluency shaping, one's mind tends to score the successes as times of fluency, and failure as moments of stuttering. This creates a situation of contradictory intention; part of you is working to be non-judgmental of moments of stuttering, while you tend to subconsciously be praising yourself for averting stuttering.*
>
> *I have seen way too many times how the same fluency strategy that "works" in practice becomes a new source of secondary tension and a sense of anticipatory anxiety when that person tries to use that tool in a real-life situation where they really want to be fluent.*

However, she added that for those who have truly overcome the need to be perfectly fluent—and are no longer concerned with the reactions of others—the use of a physical strategy to speak more fluently can be a further aspect of their empowerment. Dr. Grossman said that there are many options available, and some who play around with different stuttering modification and fluency shaping strategies discover that change is possible.

Her colleague, Carl Herder, offered this list of the potential drawbacks of fluency shaping:

1. Some people can't do fluency shaping at all outside of clinical, and everybody experiences limitations to some extent. Everyone has a moment in which they just can't do it. John

Stossel seems to be one of the few who feels so confident that he doesn't seem to have any trouble.

2. Clients who are just determined not to stutter at all tend to put up their guard more. They also practice more to ensure they feel in control.

3. Those who have had fluency shaping therapy often feel like failures or they feel guilty if they stutter, because they've been told they haven't practiced enough. But we've come to feel that this is more an indication that there is something wrong with the therapy rather than something being wrong with the client.

4. Those trained in fluency shaping sometimes don't like the way they sound when using those particular tools.

5. Fluency shaping techniques are mentally taxing, or, as speech therapists say, "high on cognitive load." We often explain this to parents by telling them to imagine trying not to use the letter "S" for an entire day. It's difficult, if not impossible, to have a spontaneous conversation while doing that, and it eliminates having authentic connections with others. It takes so much mental energy to stay perfectly on target that you can't communicate, ask good questions, or be a good listener because you are so focused on not making a mistake yourself.

6. The inherent message of fluency shaping is that fluency is good, and stuttering is bad, and we see that as a problem philosophically. It sends the client who stutters the message that there is something wrong with them. This is particularly hard on young people who want to please their friends and speech therapists, and don't want to be perceived as different from their peers.

7. We've met countless adults who tell us that they avoided stuttering by switching out words or using other methods, because they took fluency shaping training and did well in a clinical setting…but found that they still stuttered in real life.

Decide What Works Best For You

As Dr. Grossman often says, people achieve success in different ways, and they define success in different ways. Some of those who stutter are able to feel good about themselves and speak freely, even though they stutter now and then. They would rather be able to speak spontaneously without constantly feeling they are treading a minefield. They experience a big shift in perspective, from worrying about stuttering all the time to just thinking about the subject at hand and offering their thoughts without worrying if they stutter.

Others are not at all comfortable in speaking with a stutter. They are driven to be perfectly fluent. So, they spend many hours practicing the techniques taught in fluency shaping therapy. I am one of those who want to be perfect in their speech, and as a result, I can be very hard on myself if I stutter. That said, I have built a successful life with that perspective and the determination and drive it taught me.

I wouldn't say that this rigorous method is for everyone. It is, however, an option that has worked for me and many others. My fluency shaping training at Hollins under Dr. Webster changed my life. AIS is also a wonderful place that helps many, many people, and though they aren't as big on fluency shaping therapy, they sometimes do use elements of it in combination with other methods.

Every person who stutters has to decide what works best for them. My goal with this chapter and this entire book is simply to present you with a good sampling of all the therapies available to you.

6

Meditation and Mindfulness Aren't Just for Monks

There was a time when I thought meditation was just for yogis, monks, and maybe members of psychedelic sixties rock bands. Then my son, Jonathon, who was a Zen Buddhist monk for a while, suggested that meditation could help ease my anxiety over stuttering.

Jonathon is a free spirit, but also a hard worker and a very successful entrepreneur. After earning college degrees in religious studies and playwriting, he moved to Asheville, North Carolina. There, in 2001, he launched a speechwriting and leadership development service for corporate executives. He also has written three books on leadership and creativity.

Then, from 2013 to 2019, Jonathon had a very successful business that rode the wave of interest in more natural and local food products. His company, Farm to Home Milk, delivered dairy products and other goods to commercial and residential customers in the Asheville area.

Somehow, while working and raising two children, Ren and Eve, with his wife Tami, my son also found time to become a student of Zen Buddhism. He studied under Zen masters in North Carolina for more than ten years before becoming ordained as a Soto Zen Monk in 2011. So, he practices Zen and Judaism, "honoring both," as he says.

Meditation and mindfulness are major components of Zen Buddhism. Jonathon worked to become skilled at both. He even operates a meditation center called the Asheville Tiny Temple.

About ten years ago, I visited Jonathon in Asheville, and talked to him about it. Then, more recently, I saw him again after I'd attended a convention for those who stutter, and learned that meditation and mindfulness are considered very helpful therapies.

So, I asked my son to teach me the basics. I'm sure he was a little shocked, but, you know, I believe even old dogs can learn new tricks. I am always willing to try out new ways to alleviate my anxiety over stuttering, which persists even though I've managed to rise above the challenges.

Jonathon told me that one never stops practicing meditation and mindfulness, even as a Zen master. This appealed to me, since I never stop practicing methods for overcoming stuttering. He gave me instructions on meditation, teaching me to sit with my back and spine straight, my ears in line with my shoulders, and to control my breathing through my nose.

Jonathon taught me to focus on my breathing with my eyes directed at the floor, either closed or just open a little.

"Don't worry about your thoughts, just focus on your breathing," he told me.

He stressed that there is no need to worry about random thoughts and feelings coming and going during meditation. The idea is to accept they are present but not to make judgments about them or try to stop them. The approach is helpful with stuttering, since most of us with speaking challenges tend to focus on it so much that we get anxious, which can make things worse.

Mindfulness, my son said, is about letting things happen rather than fighting them, which can be applied to stuttering, too. Many times, we get so caught up in *not* stuttering that we do it more. But when we stop trying to fix it, our speech often flows much more fluently.

I tend to be very hard on myself when I stutter. I'm just one of those people who wants to be perfect in everything I do. And, since I was bullied as a child and even sometimes treated badly as an adult because of my stutter, I really am driven to speak without stuttering.

My son compared me to Sisyphus, who—according to Greek mythology—spent eternity trying to roll a giant bolder up a hill. It seemed stuttering has been my boulder, my greatest challenge. Jonathon said that mediation might help me be gentler with and more accepting of myself, which is a good thing. My son said I can still work on techniques to achieve fluent speech, but I don't have to beat myself up so much when fluency isn't attainable.

Thank goodness that Jonathon is a patient man. He taught me the basics of meditation, but like anything, it takes practice. Relaxing and clearing my mind doesn't come natural to me. I'm always juggling a dozen projects, making new plans, and am in constant motion. I had to work on the techniques and mental approaches quite a bit to get it down.

Eventually, I learned how to calm my mind and body. Everyone has to find what works best for them. I'll never be able to meditate at the level of a maharishi or a monk, but I have found a method that helps considerably.

These days I meditate on a regular basis, including right before public speaking engagements, my radio shows, big meetings, and even telephone conference calls.

I have to tell you, meditation really does help reduce my anxiety about stuttering, which in turn, along with my other work, helps me speak more fluently.

The Difference Between Meditation and Mindfulness

Meditation and mindfulness are now widely practiced in corporate America and around the world. My version of these therapies for stuttering is very simple and very effective, though maybe not as easy to do properly as you might think.

I take a few minutes to meditate by clearing my mind of all distractions. I do this by practicing breathing exercises that slow down my heart rate. I then focus my thinking on memories or images that make me feel peaceful and secure.

This is the simple way that I clear my mind for meditation. I hold my favorite pen in my hand. Put both feet flat on the ground. Close my eyes. Take slow breaths in and out. And then I think about all the stuff I've written with that pen. This clears my mind and relaxes me. Yes, this works for me. All you have to do is figure out what works for you.

Meditation is considered the formal practice of mindfulness, according to the speech therapists at AIS, who incorporate both meditation and mindfulness into their programs that use a combination of therapeutic approaches.

"We like it for a thousand reasons, and it comes up constantly in our therapy," Carl Herder of AIS told me.

He notes that the experience of stuttering is heavily influenced by the self-judgments made by those who stutter. Mindfulness and meditation help foster a "calm awareness" of what is happening inside the mind and outside the body.

"We taught this in therapy for years without ever calling it mindfulness," Carl added.

Speech therapists coached clients to pay attention to their thoughts and gestures, and especially any urge to avoid speaking or saying certain words, and to record those notes in a journal. While they tell them the goal isn't to limit those behaviors, just by noticing and noting what they are doing, they tend to do just that.

"By bringing ourselves into mind and body, we act more in line with our values," Carl explained to me. "So, if a person does not want to stutter, they focus on the behavior they don't like and do it less. Mindfulness makes you more aware of what you are doing and helps you break automatic patterns."

Mindfulness can be described simply as paying attention— without analyzing or judging—to what is going on around you and within you, whether it is the cool air coming from the air-conditioning vent, the sound of birds singing outside your window, or the thoughts running through your mind in any given moment.

Speech pathologists and researchers in the field have found that mindfulness and meditation can be transformative for those whose stutter. While they warn that it is not a cure-all, there are many who believe the benefits are considerable and maybe even "life-changing."

Letting Go and Entering the Flow

Paul Brocklehurst, a speech therapist who stutters and has a PhD in psycholinguistics, runs the Stammering Self-Empowerment Programme, a not-for-profit organization in England. He began stuttering at the age of three. As a teenager his stuttering became more severe, and when he started working towards a medical degree at university, it became so severe that he found it impossible to continue and finally dropped out.

After leaving medical school, he grew depressed and went through "a dark night of the soul," as he later wrote in a highly regarded essay, "Mindfulness and Stuttering."

But then, at the age of twenty, he read the 1974 classic book on meditation *Zen and the Art of Motorcycle Maintenance*. It inspired him to do more research on meditation and mindfulness, reading more books and delving into the science behind them. He ultimately joined a Zen group where he became a devoted practitioner of meditation, sitting formally for two or three hours a day and making effort to remain mindful while performing actions throughout the remainder of the day.

After a year and a half, he realized that his stutter had all but disappeared. Brocklehurst and most other researchers in his field believe his case was extraordinary. He attributes his improvement to a combination of factors, including not just the meditation and mindfulness, but also the major lifestyle changes that he adopted in order to be allowed to join the Zen group. Some years later, when he finally left the Zen group and adopted a more worldly lifestyle, some minor symptoms of stuttering returned.

Most people who stutter won't lose theirs entirely. Still, speech therapists say meditation can be an effective tool for those who use it effectively and spend significant time doing it.

Experts point to a 2012 study in which participants found that mindfulness and meditation reduced the impact of stuttering on their lives and helped them stutter less frequently. Being mindful helps ease the tension over the fear of stuttering, increasing awareness of the presence of negative thoughts cycling through the mind.

When those who stutter realize these thoughts are present, they can disarm them, distancing themselves from those crippling thoughts and emotions. Letting go of the fear of stuttering, which allows you to stop fighting it or trying to fix it, relieves a lot of the pressure as you speak. "It turned my life around. It was the first time I'd ever really been able to enjoy life," Brocklehurst said in a 2017 interview with a Headspace.com blogger.

In his noted essay on mindfulness and stuttering, he describes two types of mindfulness: (1) passively observing where your attention is currently going and (2) actively trying to focus your attention on something in particular.

Dr. Brocklehurst makes a point to also say that mindfulness is not a form of relaxation. Instead, it is about being aware if you feel relaxed, or stressed, or angry—and open to the experience, whatever it might be. It also is not a process for "emptying" your mind of thoughts. Instead, it helps you learn to control how much attention you pay to your thoughts.

Mindfulness is a useful tool for those who stutter because "it can help us identify exactly what we do when we stutter," he writes in the essay. Speech therapists can use mindfulness to train those who stutter to identify the behaviors that are involved, including the entire sensory experience—body language, facial movements, interrupted speech flow, and listener response.

Dr. Brocklehurst said mindfulness also helps those who stutter avoid paying attention to value judgments about the quality of their speech. This is good, because when we feel our fluency isn't good enough, it puts pressure on us to do better and makes us anxious.

Although he admits it isn't always easy to do, Brocklehurst advises us to avoid judging our speech and to stay in the moment, focusing on the experience without rating it good or bad. "Remember, the more you focus on the raw experiences, the less space there is for your mind to make such judgments," he writes in the essay.

Mainstream Mindfulness and Meditation

Even Fortune 500 companies like General Mills, Goldman Sachs, Google, Apple, and Nike encourage their employees to practice mindfulness, and some have classes on site. This makes sense when you consider that mindfulness is helpful in focusing your attention, controlling responses to emotions, reducing stress, alleviating anxiety, and relieving milder forms of depression.

Dr. Brocklehurst attests that practicing mindfulness has proven to be life-changing for many who stutter. AIS team members say their clients often have found that it helps increase overall awareness of both body and mind, allowing them to pause, pick up on speech patterns, and make decisions on their responses during communication.

As with most therapeutic approaches, no one method works for everyone. Fortunately, there are many approaches to practicing mindfulness. I've used several of them myself. Here are four popular methods that have been tried by clients under the guidance of the AIS philosophy.

Breath Awareness

Sit with your back straight and eyes closed. Pay attention to the flow of your breathing in and out and how it feels in your nose, chest, or belly. Your mind will wander; that's okay. The idea is to pay attention and keep refocusing on your breathing. They say every time your mind wanders and you bring it back, you actually get better at focusing, so consider it part of the process to learn mindfulness. Take it one breath at a time, staying focused on the present. Try to do this for ten minutes at least once or twice a day.

Body Scan

This method is designed to help you develop a sense of the mind and body connection, and to guide you in checking in on your body and how it's functioning. There's no judgment or need to change anything; rather, you're just bringing attention to each part of your body and noting how each part is connected to the next. You might want to envision yourself in a hospital body scanner, watching as it scans from your head down through your torso and to your feet. As it scans, be aware of any tension points or tightness you feel during the sequence.

Monitor your thoughts and feelings and whether you're comfortable or restless, again without trying to change or fix anything. Just pay attention and monitor your breathing as the scan progresses down and then back up. Notice how everything is connected, even how your skin feels around your body as your chest and stomach expand and contract as you breathe.

Self-Compassion

This is a big one for me, because, as I've said before, I tend to get down on myself when I'm not speaking as fluently as I want. This is true of many of us who stutter—we are often kinder and more understanding to other people than we are to ourselves. That's why practicing mindful self-compassion is highly recommended by the speech therapists at AIS.

When you catch yourself being self-critical or judgmental, stop and ask whether you would treat a friend the same way. There are meditations that encourage self-compassion specifically. These follow the usual steps for meditation while including reminders to be kind and compassionate to yourself, aiming to be as accepting of yourself as you would be of a friend.

RAIN Meditation

RAIN stands for Recognizing, Allowing, Investigating, and Nurturing, which is a process for dealing with difficult emotions. Those who stutter deal with many negative feelings, including frustration, anger, sadness, humiliation, and anxiety. The RAIN meditations provide a healthy way to deal with those emotions instead of venting them, or turning to alcohol, drugs, over-eating, or other unhealthy distractions.

The Benefits of Calm Awareness

Mindfulness helps you create a calm awareness of whatever is occurring in each moment, both inside your mind and body and all around you. Again, the idea isn't to judge anything or anyone, but to simply notice it.

AIS speech therapists say this can be helpful to those of us who stutter, allowing us to be aware of tension in our bodies and negative thoughts playing out in our minds. Meditation helps in the practice of flexing the mindfulness muscle in preparation for those difficult stuttering moments. The concept is simple, but learning to make it a habit—especially during moments of stuttering—can be a challenge. AIS speech therapists offer this guidance to those seeking to be more mindful by trying meditation:

Don't worry about becoming a master of meditation or perfect at it according to some set standards. Instead, be open to whatever works for you, and be patient with your efforts to learn what that might be. Accept that you won't feel comfortable and successful at first. It's all about trying and learning from failures.

Falling asleep is not a sign of failure. For some, that's a goal. If you don't want to fall asleep, try meditating at a time of day when you have the most energy, like first thing in the morning.

Your style of meditation may not be like anyone else's. We all have our unique styles of walking, talking, and engaging with the world, so that's okay. There are people who can meditate while hiking in the woods—good for them! And good for you, no matter what methods work best! Using a meditation guide or class can be a helpful way to get started. Some people always use a guide or a partner. There are many resources online, too.

The Power to Choose

These tools and techniques can be very helpful, because they put you in control. You can choose how you respond to negative thoughts and tensions in your body, instead of letting them control you and impacting your ability to communicate.

Consider taking a class or joining a group to learn meditation and mindfulness techniques. This will get you off to a faster start. Classes are easy to find these days, and many corporations and fitness centers offer them. General classes won't be custom designed for those who stutter, but once you've mastered the basics, you can adjust for your specific needs, as I have.

Ending the Shame Game

Many people who stutter have benefitted from meditation and mindfulness, and some have gone on to become strong advocates of this form of therapy. Samantha "Sam" Gennuso wrote a compelling story featured on the AIS website in January 2020 about her many years of torment with a covert stutter. She hid her stutter as a teen and self-medicated with alcohol in her twenties.

Now a "pre-licensed psychotherapist" and recovery coach, she credits meditation and mindfulness for helping her heal. She writes:

Stuttering was a foreign concept to me, because I didn't let myself audibly block. My shame about what it meant to stutter, the physical reactions my body had endured over years of fight/ flight/freeze and hyper vigilance, anticipation and low self-esteem in stark contrast to the high expectations of others, would follow me through college and into my twenties where I would discover that alcohol and other substances substantially numbed the feeling of failure as an identity that stuttering had imprinted on my psyche.

She noted that becoming aware of internal, unconscious reactions to stuttering and the related shame that manifests is vital for healing and recovering. For many of those who stutter, shame is a constant challenge, Sam said.

She and many others have found that mindfulness practices help them "by rewiring neuropathways and recalibrating the autonomic nervous system."

"Recent research shows us that yoga, meditation and breathwork can actually change the way we react physically to different stressors and triggers. This can literally change the manifestation of stuttering in the voice and body," she wrote on the AIS website.

Below is a list of resources for guided meditation that the AIS recommends for its clients, passed on to you with their permission. They are not specifically designed for people who stutter, but can be helpful for those wanting to practice mindfulness.

Jon Kabat-Zinn: Body Scan

This is helpful for first-timers. Jon Kabat-Zinn is an American professor emeritus of medicine and the creator of the Stress Reduction Clinic and the Center for Mindfulness in Medicine, Health Care, and Society at the University of Massachusetts Medical School. He asks you to lie down and takes you through a thirty-minute body scan. It is very relaxing but try to stay awake! (Good luck with that.)

Jonathan Foust

Jonathan Foust is a guiding teacher with the Insight Meditation Community of Washington and a founder of the Meditation Teacher Training Institute in Washington. AIS speech therapists recommend his *Energy Awareness Meditations* CD and streaming audio, and his website (www.jonathanfoust.com), which provides a twenty-minute guided meditation as well as several podcasts.

Guided Meditation Apps Available on iTunes and Google Play

Insight Timer: Meditation App

This app has a lot of free content and builds a sense of community.

Calm: Meditation to Relax, Focus, and Sleep Better

Free content and a large library of meditations with a paid monthly membership. You can select background sounds and imagery like babbling brooks, fireplaces, rainforests, and beach sunsets. There is also a good introduction to daily meditation with a seven-day program.

10% Happier

Apple's Best of 2018 app is helpful for learning to meditate, sleep better, and be happier. It comes from author and former *Good Morning America* correspondent Dan Harris, who wrote a book of the same name.

Buddhify: Modern Mindfulness for Busy Lives

This five-dollar app provides guided meditations for life activities.

The Mindfulness App: Meditation for Everyone

Offers free and paid options that are great for beginners and advanced meditation, too.

Sitting Still

Aimed at teens and offers a mix of free and paid guided meditations.

Headspace

Offers both free content and an optional monthly membership with a cool buddy system option to share with friends. Has a cartoonish style that is appealing and has a website article discussing meditation and stuttering.

Omvana: Meditation for Everyone

This app allows for customized meditation and provides information on several meditation experts.

7

A Holistic Approach Offers a Deeper Dive into Speech Therapy

Jeremiah Kitchen isn't one of those librarians who will "shush" those who speak up in his realm. After nearly three decades of silencing himself because of a severe stutter, he now revels in communicating with his library patrons—and even complete strangers.

"I had developed a lifestyle of silence, of solitude, of fear, and of repressing my true personality," he recalled in an AIS blog. "All of my speech-therapy in the past had 'failed,' even to the point of making my speech worse, not better."

The quality of Jeremiah's life changed dramatically for the better after he attended an AIS three-week intensive therapy program at the age of thirty. Upon completion of the program, he returned home to Denver and continued bi-weekly and then monthly therapy on Skype for the next three years.

The difference in this program was that it was a more holistic approach that addressed the deeper problems behind his stuttering through several methods, including cognitive behavioral retraining, he said.

"The clinicians and I worked together to examine and modify what I believed about stuttering, how I felt about stuttering and what I did or didn't do in response to stuttering—or to my fear of stuttering," Jeremiah said.

Free to Be Yourself

Jeremiah benefitted greatly from cognitive restructuring.

"I stutter still, but in a different way, to where the interruptions in my speech don't interfere much with my communication," he writes. "In addition, (and this is the most important part), my overall well-being has increased, and I do not avoid speaking or speaking situations because of stuttering. In short: I no longer let stuttering restrict my participation in life. This, I believe, is the criteria by which 'successful' treatment for stuttering should be judged."

Jeremiah said that between the ages of eighteen and thirty he rarely spoke to anyone. The holistic approach has given him the confidence to do many things he'd previously avoided. He now enjoys offering his point of view in conversations, taking the initiative to meet new people and talking on the telephone.

"It took me a long time to feel comfortable with my voice, to not hate it and not fear it, but to use it freely and fully," he said.

Changing the Mindset

While fluency shaping and stuttering modification emphasize physically retraining the client's speech, cognitive behavioral retraining focuses more on changing the mindset that feeds fear in those who stutter, Dr. Grossman noted in our discussions.

Through cognitive behavioral retraining, clients learn how their inner thoughts contribute to their emotions, and how this impacts their physical stuttering. Then, they work on disputing and shifting these thoughts by going out and completing speaking challenges in the real world to support their new, healthier thoughts and behavior.

Every speech therapist might have his or her own definition of holistic therapy, which is an integrated approach that might include affective behavioral cognitive change, stuttering modification, and fluency shaping. For example, the AIS intense therapy program that helped Jeremiah is custom designed for each individual, and also often incorporates avoidance reduction, self-disclosure, voluntary stuttering, mindfulness meditation, somatic therapy, and support with others who stutter.

"The holistic approach includes addressing feelings and attitudes, what we call the 'ABC's of stuttering,' which refers to the affective, behavioral, and cognitive aspects," Carl Herder told me.

Carl and his colleagues think of the holistic approach as stuttering therapy that addresses their clients' daily experiences as people who stutter.

"We are emotional beings and we thrive when connecting with others," Carl explained in our interviews. "We have a varying set of emotions that we experience around people, and holistic stuttering therapy takes all of that into account. We look at what it is like for a person who stutters to experience stuttering and find ways to help them manage it in real life, not just in the vacuum of a clinical study."

In this manner, holistic approaches address the affective, behavioral, and cognitive aspects of stuttering with an individualized approach that helps most people make sustainable change.

"We try to remove a lot of the things that can create cognitive dissonance, such as the seemingly conflicting practices of advising clients to accept that they stutter while also teaching them ways to be more fluent," said Carl.

Treating the Emotional Turmoil Caused by Stuttering

In the past, speech therapists at AIS and other treatment centers had used a "toolbox" or "smorgasbord" approach that taught some fluency techniques and some methods for reducing tension in moments of stuttering, as well as some voluntary stuttering and ways to accept inevitable moments of stuttering.

The rationale, back then, was to let clients experience a variety of techniques and choose those that worked best for them. The problem with that blend of approaches was that some of them seemed to conflict with others, which, understandably, confused people.

In the AIS intensive therapy programs, there was a strong focus on emotional and cognitive factors, in addition to the physical aspects of stuttering. Their therapists found that by the end of the three-week program, most clients were using specific speech skills to speak more fluently, and often said they were more confident in communicating.

But then, many clients began reporting that they weren't able to maintain their level of fluency over time. Their fear of speaking and avoidance behaviors returned. Some returned for refresher programs. Clients said they felt guilty or ashamed, or even hopeless because their stuttering had returned. Because of these negative feelings, they'd begun to avoid specific words or speaking in public.

In response, AIS began intensive programs that were more individualized and based on each client's experience, values, and learning styles. The programs still were based on successful and proven treatment methods designed to reduce fears of stuttering and maximize communications skills, encouraging the client to speak openly and confidently whether stuttering or not.

One of the goals was to help clients become "fluent" in stuttering by reducing avoidance behaviors, physical struggles, and fears in their daily lives.

"We found that when we talked to speech therapists working in schools, they felt that most of those speech tools involving fluency shaping and stuttering modification were frustrating for them and the students they worked with. Often, they would lose their direction," Carl told me.

The school speech therapists wanted to find ways to help their students. Their input lead to the development of the holistic approach, or integrated therapy, which involves the following:

1. Reducing negative emotional responses, by talking about stuttering.
2. Reducing avoidance behaviors, which can involve different ways to distract from stuttering, escape from it, or to avoid it before it happens.

3. Enhancing overall communication skills including eye contact, intonation, projecting, posture, asking good questions, and active listening.

4. Environmental management, support, and learning to self-advocate. This involves learning how to educate your friends about stuttering, so you are more willing to talk about it with them. It can also include checking in with teachers to make sure you will not be penalized for stuttering, letting people know you will stutter when you meet them, and making sure co-workers understand stuttering.

5. Reducing the physical struggle of stuttering by stuttering forward, letting the stutter happen and moving through it rather than waiting for the "magic moment" when all of a sudden, the word comes out. A lot of speakers wait for that moment, and the waiting gets reinforced so much that it becomes part of the pattern of stuttering.

"We encourage people to stutter their way through, as opposed to postponing it or waiting it out," Carl explained in our interviews. "Some push way harder than they need to, which can result in really tense vocal struggle. They are straining their voices more than they need to. They can learn to speak without so much struggle, but that involves a lot of exploration."

Jeremiah benefitted from the holistic approach, which made a dramatic change in his life. He said that the holistic program differed from other therapies because "it addressed more than just the surface behaviors of stuttering."

This approach helped identify "the source of the real problem," which, in Jeremiah's case, was "(mostly) [his] over-reactive and maladaptive reactions to stuttering," he wrote.

Jeremiah noted that he and the clinicians worked together to examine and modify:

1. What he believed about stuttering
2. How he felt about stuttering
3. What he did or didn't do in response to stuttering, or the fear of stuttering

The process is neither fast nor easy. In an article written for the AIS website in 2015, Jeremiah offered that it requires much time, analysis, confrontation, and courage. But this deeper dive into stuttering therapy has opened a new chapter in the librarian's life. His stuttering has not disappeared, but it is "less abnormal, less tense and shorter in duration."

Rational Emotive Behavior Therapy

Jeremiah benefitted from another approach in the holistic toolbox known as Rational Emotive Behavior Therapy (REBT), which was created by pioneering psychologist Albert Ellis in the 1950s and served as the original cognitive behavioral therapy.

"Many clients like Jeremiah have long and elaborate histories of speech therapy that largely focused on how to be fluent. This often gave them certain core beliefs that they *should* be able to use tools, be fluent, and control their stutters," Dr. Grossman told me.

"This process increases fear of stuttering over time, which tends to make their struggles and avoidance efforts worse. REBT restructures those beliefs, and in so doing, the clients find they can accept themselves regardless of their speech. This helps them stop making undue demands on themselves that just make their stutter worse."

This form of psychotherapy is also considered a philosophy for living that has proven useful in combination with avoidance reduction, stuttering modification, and other therapies. REBT helps those who stutter identify, challenge, and change negative thoughts, feelings, and beliefs.

Dr. Grossman co-authored a notable paper on this topic with Dr. Gunars Neiders, a PhD psychologist in Washington State, who provides in-person and internet-based stuttering treatment. His website is www.stutteringrecovery.net.

As Heather and Dr. Neiders explain in the paper, "REBT is based on the premise that we do not become upset directly because of the events that happen to us. Rather, the beliefs we hold about these events cause us to become depressed, anxious, enraged, etc."

For example, if you feel someone is laughing with you, your response will be much different than if you think they are laughing at you, they note. They cite Epictetus, the Greek philosopher, as the first to articulate this nearly two thousand years ago when he said, "Men are disturbed not by events, but by the views which they take of them."

REBT approaches don't try to "overhaul" a client's speech. Instead, they work to modify the negative and intrusive thoughts that disrupt their speaking. As Dr. Grossman and Dr. Neiders describe in their paper, the goal of REBT is to achieve "free-flowing" speech, which allows you to:

- Communicate effectively, saying what you want to say, where and when you want to say it, with and without stuttering.
- Be open to self-disclose your stuttering, stutter openly, and talk about your stuttering with others in both casual and serious conversations.

- Recognize that all people have breaks in their fluency, so you shouldn't feel pressured to be perfect.
- Stutter with varying frequency and tension but always with self-dignity and confidence.
- Recognize that while you may prefer fluency, you shouldn't demand it of yourself, or put yourself down for stuttering "too much."
- Minimize avoidance behaviors and use of tricks, crutches, and efforts to push through stuttering moments. Even when you do fall into those behaviors, you will be more self-aware and able to self-correct without getting down on yourself or feeling shame.

Dr. Grossman considers REBT to be a "semantic therapy," meaning that the words we say—and even think—are critical, since they affect how we feel, think, and act. They encourage those who stutter to use words wisely in their self-communication as well as when talking to others, considering both a word's actual meaning and any connotations that derive from it.

For example, rather than thinking, *My stutter is bad today,* speech therapists would encourage you to think, *I am stuttering more today.* This reduces the negative connotations around the stutter.

This therapy also tries to free those who stutter from torturing themselves by fixating on being perfect in their speaking, or demanding that others treat them exactly as they want to be treated.

To quote the Rolling Stones, "You can't always get what you want." So, give yourself what's needed: permission to be a perfectly imperfect human being doing the best you can. Otherwise, you will be burdened with anxiety, depression, shame, guilt, self-pity, and procrastination. Speech often flows more freely if we are not focused on chasing complete fluency.

Dr. Grossman notes that when those of us who stutter worry about being bullied or laughed at, then:

- Negative emotions kick in
- We stutter more and longer
- Our secondary behaviors kick in, including blinking, finger snapping, and not maintaining eye contact

Speech therapists say the real problem isn't judgmental listeners and their responses. Instead, it's our own conviction that stuttering is bad and should be stifled entirely.

In their paper, Dr. Grossman and Dr. Neiders identify categories of "Gremlin Thoughts" that create anxiety and trigger avoidance behaviors.

1. *Self-downing.* This is a belief that if you don't live up to your goal of overcoming your stutter, you will be condemned or considered a loser.

2. *Low frustration tolerance and underestimating personal resiliency.* This is the belief that you can't stand the discomfort and frustration of experiencing stuttering, or that it would feel "too weird" to self-disclose or stutter on purpose.

3. *Awfulizing and catastrophizing.* When you exaggerate the negative aspects of stuttering or spend too much time dwelling on a stuttering moment, speech therapists call it "awfulizing" because you are letting it get to you more than you should. You may dwell on how bad you stuttered when, in reality, it wasn't that bad; conversely, you may worry about something terrible occurring if you stutter.

4. *Overgeneralizing.* This is taking things to negative extremes for no good reason, with thoughts that dwell on past failures as if they will always be repeated. One example: *I always stutter on the phone and I always will.* Another example: *I still stutter so I will never be free of it. I will always be burdened by it.*

Despite this belief, there are so many successful people in the world who have stuttered and even still stutter. Many of them I've mentioned throughout this book: Joe Biden, John Stossel, Austin Pendleton, Arthur Blank, Samuel L. Jackson, Bruce Willis, Emily Blunt, and Ed Sheeran. They are all doing just fine in life, and so can you!

5. *Shoulds, musts, and must-nots.* These are rigid demands you place on yourself, demanding that you must be fluent. They can also include self-imposed time pressures to limit your speaking. You can eliminate much of the tension of this gremlin by accepting that stuttering is permissible.

6. *Mind-reading.* This is the tendency to be overly concerned about what others will think or say if you stutter. This comes with the common assumption by those who stutter that other people don't want to listen to them speak, or others will be uncomfortable if they stutter.

When you find those emotional hot links simmering in your thoughts and stirring your negative emotions, ask yourself these questions:

- Where is the evidence that this is true?
- Does it make sense based on your real-world experiences?
- Is it helping you?

Just by asking yourself things like, "Why do I care what anyone thinks?" you shift your mindset away from negative emotions, including the need to please others or to be perfect. We are all imperfect, after all. And if someone is bothered by your stuttering, that is their problem, not yours.

Now, I know that convincing yourself of this may take some time and effort. Be as patient and compassionate toward yourself as you would be to those you care about. You have a right to be happy—don't let anyone else take that away from you.

You might find it helpful to keep a journal of your fight for self-assurance. Keep a record of all the times you have negative hot-link thoughts and then counter them with empowering words.

Dr. Grossman has also put together a list that helps her clients recognize stuttering gremlins when they enter their thoughts.

Top Ten Lies Spread by Stuttering Gremlins

1. Stuttering is an abnormality. Stuttering is *bad*. It is not something a dignified adult would do.
   YOUR ANTI-GREMLIN RESPONSE: *I'd say Emily Blunt, James Earl Jones, and former vice president Joe Biden, all of whom have stutters, qualify as dignified people, wouldn't you?*

2. People do not like talking to those who stutter. It requires too much patience, and most don't have that. They think anyone who stutters is stupid and nervous.
   YOUR ANTI-GREMLIN RESPONSE: *Jack Welch was CEO of General Electric, and when he retired, they gave him $413 million. So, I guess that wasn't because they thought he was stupid, right?*

3. When you speak, you should not take up too much time. It is wrong to make people wait for you to talk. Fast is good and slow is bad.

   YOUR ANTI-GREMLIN RESPONSE: *If I have something valuable to say, people will wait to hear it! I'm not trying to sell them a car on a television commercial, I'm communicating!*

4. Stuttering too much will keep you from having a good education, getting a good job, and having meaningful relationships with others.

   YOUR ANTI-GREMLIN RESPONSE: *Multi-billionaire Richard Branson stutters and has dyslexia, yet his Virgin Group includes more than four hundred companies. Did I mention that he and his wife, Joan Templeman, have been married more than thirty years?*

5. You should focus on speaking fluently and use whatever tactics available to you in order to avoid stuttering and to be fluent.

   YOUR ANTI-GREMLIN RESPONSE: *Sorry, goofy Gremlin, the AIS philosophy holds that chasing fluency is not the answer. But if you can learn to relax and calm yourself, your stutter will not be a burden to you.*

6. It is better not to speak, or to enter situations that may expose you as a person who stutters.

   YOUR ANTI-GREMLIN RESPONSE: *Tell that to Bruce Willis, Samuel L. Jackson, and Tiger Woods! They have all talked openly about stuttering and how they've overcome any fears of speaking in public.*

7. Stuttering is a shameful topic and it is better to keep it to yourself.

    YOUR ANTI-GREMLIN RESPONSE: *See my response in No. 6! Are you paying attention, Gremlins?*

8. Even if you have something good to say, stuttering will diminish it.

    YOUR ANTI-GREMLIN RESPONSE: *Have you ever heard the "Iron Curtain" speech? Historians say it is one of the most inspiring speeches in history. It was given by Sir Winston Churchill, who stuttered and had a lisp.*

9. Life would be so much better if you could control your stuttering.

    YOUR ANTI-GREMLIN RESPONSE: *First of all, Gremlin dude, speaking isn't about control, it's about being free and open and relaxed! And if you think Pulitzer Prize-winning rapper Kendrick Lamar and Grammy-winning singer Ed Sheeran don't enjoy their lives, well, you may need to take your Gremlin brain in for a tune-up.*

10. It is more important to say something fluently than risk saying what you really want to say and stuttering.

    YOUR ANTI-GREMLIN RESPONSE: *Read this book's next chapter on the power of public speaking! Do you think Capt. Sully worried about his stutter when he told his flight controllers that he was landing his passenger plane on the Hudson River? Wrong again on No. 10, Gremlin!*

You Can Live Fully with Stuttering

According to Dr. Grossman, REBT builds unconditional self-acceptance whether or not you stutter. "You don't need to change a single thing except your attitude," she writes in the paper with Dr. Neiders. "Self-acceptance is available to you no matter what, even when you behave foolishly, and no matter how severely you stutter. You simply choose to accept yourself and nothing else is required."

Here are examples of unconditional self-acceptance, a process where you actively acknowledge that you don't have to be perfect. They were included in the paper by Dr. Grossman and Dr. Neiders:

- *I am a fallible human being; I have my good points and my bad points.*
- *There is no reason why I must not have flaws.*
- *Despite my good points and my bad points, I am no more worthy and no less worthy than any other human being.*

By keeping rational messages like these in mind to fend off negative and self-defeating thoughts, you can build yourself up, acting on positive self-talk to achieve self-respect and dignity.

"You cannot expect another person to respect you if you do not treat yourself with respect," these two veteran speech therapists write in their paper. "If you feel you are not being treated with dignity, you need to be willing to stand up for yourself."

Dr. Grossman and Dr. Neiders encourage clients to never apologize for stuttering, but to instead stutter with confidence, maintaining normal eye contact and social contact with whomever you are speaking to. You should feel free to make requests, such as: *"Hello, I have a speech impediment. I stutter, so please be patient as it will take me some extra time to speak."*

Other suggestions from the speech pathologist and the psychologist who specialize in stuttering therapies include:

- Instead of resenting that you have to self-disclose, feeling it is something you are giving the other person, try recalling that self-disclosure allows you to stutter freely. Feel proud of how you disclose with confidence, even though it's not always easy.
- Instead of condemning yourself for stuttering with tension, try giving yourself credit for saying what you want to say, especially since it may result in more stuttering. Remind yourself that you are resilient.
- Instead of beating yourself up for avoiding a word or situation, try using the fact that you now have the awareness that these behaviors are not helpful as a positive reminder of how far you've come.
- Instead of feeling bad because you let yourself get embarrassed that you stuttered, try having pride that you pushed through discomfort. You made eye contact even though you were uncomfortable stuttering.

Dr. Grossman tells me that REBT really helps people make progress changing their avoidance behaviors by altering the underlying thoughts that precipitate their avoidance efforts.

"We also greatly emphasize desensitization, mindfulness practices, and developing skills for increasing overall communicative effectiveness. Again, we find REBT helps people increase their readiness and ability to complete these challenges," she said.

Now, as Dr. Grossman has noted, sometimes the best self-talk and emotional state alone do not change the stubborn habits of forcing and struggling with our speech. There is a learned motor component to stuttering that is akin to a habit—and habit forma-tion can play a big role, she said. Reactions to moments of stuttering can become habitual, including physical movements:

In such cases, REBT will help reduce the thoughts and emotions that trigger the habit. Working on stuttering more easily and with more confidence—along with practicing some voluntary stuttering—can help reduce that habitual muscle memory.

This type of holistic treatment can also work with avoid-ance behavior reduction and "safety behaviors," such as leaving a group of people to avoid introductions or texting instead of talking on the telephone. "REBT harmonizes so well with avoid-ance reduction while recognizing that we all have to choose our battles," she explained. "In my opinion, if a safety behavior is only occasional and not self-defeating, it can be just fine to have some self-acceptance without putting yourself down for making it easier on yourself."

REBT Helps Children Who Stutter

Dr. Grossman recommends the use of REBT for children as well as adults who stutter. She notes that the foundation of REBT, whether applied to stuttering or in any other area of human behavior, is—above all else—to influence the client to understand that the goal is to live fully. You and I do not have to prove to anyone, including ourselves, that we are good, or fluent, or able to achieve free-flow-ing speech.

"These ideas really do translate nicely to work with children," Dr. Grossman said. "I find that even very young children come to therapy already having constructed that stuttering is 'bad' and that they are being 'good' when they do something that prevents a stutter."

When working with children, they often tell her that what bothers them most about stuttering is usually the fear of being teased or laughed at. REBT therapy teaches us that wanting approval and fair treatment is only human, but the reactions of others don't really matter all that much. Those who stutter can't let other people and their judgments stop us from living freely and chasing our dreams. The only thing that matters is what we think of ourselves—and holistic therapies such as REBT help us remember to be our own best friends and encouragers.

AIS speech therapists work to help children learn that *all* people have their strengths and flaws and that they make us uniquely human and amazing, Dr. Grossman explained:

> We emphasize that the most important thing about communication is to use it to interact with others and to get things done—saying exactly what you want to say—stutter or not. As listeners, we send that message by reinforcing content, listening actively, and interacting genuinely, not by reinforcing fluent speech.

8

Public Speaking Won't Kill You; It May Even Help You!

For most of us who stutter, the thought of giving a speech seems more like a torture than a treatment. Yet, speech therapists and other experts tell me that public speaking has proven to be very therapeutic for those who've learned techniques for reducing anxiety and conquering their fears.

You can take heart in the fact that those of us who stutter are not alone in our fear of public speaking. It is one of the most common of all fears. Twenty-five percent of the general population are believed to share that dread, according to a 2015 article on the website of PsychologyToday.com. This fear is even stronger among those of us who stutter. Believe me, I know. I've had to give countless speeches over the years in my PR and marketing career. Even today, I often speak to groups and I have a weekly radio show on public service radio called *Leader's Edge*.

Despite all of the speeches and radio shows I have done over the years, my heart still starts pumping faster when I step up to a microphone or a podium. Yet, here I am recommending that you do all the public speaking you can handle, because it has proven to be a great therapy for people like you and me.

Carl Herder has seen many clients derive great benefits from public speaking workshops as part of a combination of therapies. "Some even transition into improv workshops and join the Toastmasters public speaking organization because their confidence is so much greater," Carl said.

Stepping Up and Speaking Up

Carl's client, Dhruva Kathuria, the doctoral student at Texas A&M, is among those who've benefitted from stepping up and speaking up at Toastmasters events. The international organization, which has chapters in 143 countries, provides public speaking and leadership training for members as well as opportunities to hone their speaking skills at events.

Dhruva—who struggled from childhood with his stutter, but has improved dramatically through avoidance reduction and voluntary stuttering therapies—joined Toastmasters in Texas. In an interview for the book, Dhruva said he signed up in the fall semester at Texas A&M and signed up to speak at the first meeting because "[he] knew the longer [he] waited to give [his] speech, the tougher it would get."

For someone who had become very skilled at avoiding speaking in his younger years, Dhruva made a brave choice for his first speech. His topic was stuttering. He talked about its impact on his life and how he'd come to feel it had made him a stronger person.

"The speech went well, and I had a lot of people congratulating me and telling me that it was one of the best first speeches they had heard. I was on cloud nine, honestly," he said. "I think Toastmasters is a different experience than my normal talks at conferences, because I know the material better at the conferences since that's what I have been doing my research on for so many years now. So, I am in general more confident."

His fellow Toastmasters members provide feedback on eye contact and body language, as well as the way speakers move and present themselves. Dhruva found it nerve-wracking at first, but helpful in the long run.

"It was tough, but also a great learning experience to understand that a good talk goes way beyond fluency," he said.

Toastmasters challenges its members to give impromptu speeches to each other, and to evaluate each other, which Dhruva said can be tough for someone who stutters. Though, he also explains "it makes you take on your fears week after week, and also forces you to focus on other aspects of your talk such as smiling, pausing, and making eye contact. So it can be rewarding, for sure."

Dhruva found it also helped him to learn that even people who don't stutter are "scared as hell" to stand up on stage and talk. "Frankly, I have never understood why people who speak fluently are so scared," he said. "What's the worst that can happen to them?"

Carl gave him a good example of the difference between public speaking for a person who stutters versus a person who speaks without a stutter. "He said running a marathon is very difficult for a person with a prosthetic leg, but that doesn't make it any easier for the person with two good legs," Dhruva said.

Dhruva did have some advice for others who stutter and are considering joining a group like Toastmasters. He suggested that they join only after they are comfortable self-advertising, facing their fears, and accepting their stuttering. He actually tried to join Toastmasters twice—once in India and once after coming to the U.S.—but those attempts were before his AIS therapy with Carl, when his "old stuttering beliefs" were still too powerful.

"I attended the first meeting and just sat there frozen in my seat, because the panic induced by the thought of going on stage was too strong," Dhruva recalled. It was only after his sessions at AIS that he was able to engage fully with Toastmasters, because he'd become more accepting of his stutter and more willing to speak openly.

"I wouldn't dive right into it without being at that point, because it could have the opposite effect on you if you are not ready for so much public speaking," he said. "If a person who stutters has not faced stuttering in less challenging situations, then going on stage could do more harm than good."

He suggested that those who stutter join Toastmasters only if they've worked on developing a healthy mindset, warning that otherwise, you can fall into the trap of comparing yourself to other speakers in the organization who don't have to manage stutters:

For a person who stutters, speech is tied to self-worth, and such comparisons can cause a lot of pain. I have done this myself as well. So, it is essential to remind yourself that you are there to improve as a communicator and not to compare or compete with others.

Toastmasters is not a means to eliminate or "fix" your stuttering, Dhruva stressed. But if you are ready to step up and speak out to improve your communication skills, go for it. "You are a person who stutters and there is a chance that you will stutter on stage. It will be tough to experience for sure, but you will be fine," he said. "Don't put an unreasonable expectation on yourself to be fluent, and lastly, enjoy."

Prepping for the Podium

As terrifying as speaking to large groups may seem to those who stutter, I do believe that facing that fear and making speeches has benefitted me over the years. My confidence has grown with every speech, and that has kept me motivated to practice my techniques for speaking more fluently.

Stepping up to speak to an audience is still not easy, I'll give you that. But if you master techniques that are taught by speech therapists like those at HCRI and AIS, you will find that public speaking can be very therapeutic. You will feel more confident and comfortable in day-to-day conversations, even if you trip up on words now and then.

I've developed a practice routine before I give a speech or do a radio show. I practice breathing through my nose to calm myself. I take slow, comfortable, full breaths. I also practice slowing down as I speak to prepare for those words that are speed bumps for me—those with hard letters, including the Gs, Bs, and Ds.

When I'm writing a speech, I make notes within it reminding myself to take full breaths and change the tempo, pause, and contour the amplitude by beginning each sound softly and building from there on initial sounds like G, B, D, or S.

For big speeches, I often have a teleprompter, so I can read directly from it with those notes included. Then, when I step up to the podium, I remind myself to take my time and not rush. I usually mark up my speeches with breaks, a method also used by England's King George VI, whose stuttering challenges were featured in the Academy Award-winning movie *The King's Speech*.

The point is that you can give a great speech even if you stutter, so don't let your fears keep you off the podium.

One thing to note about public speaking fears is that, while they are common, if you think your fear goes beyond what is normal, you should talk to a mentor, psychologist, or psychiatrist. I mention this because there is a condition called social anxiety disorder, which produces a higher level of distress when interacting with others. There are treatments for it as well, but they are more sophisticated than those for the usual public speaking anxieties.

By the way, I think it's sort of a cruel joke that the scientific name for the fear of public speaking is glossophobia, which would trip off anyone's tongue! So, I suppose it is not a coincidence that the term is derived from the Greek words for "tongue" and "fear."

Practice, Practice, Practice

Practice is important—whether you are giving a speech or playing a sport or an instrument—but it is even more critical for the public speaker with a stutter. We have to be disciplined to put in the extra effort in preparing for a speech, which is something my mother reminded me all of my life.

Admittedly, my methods for preparing a public speech are more hardcore than those recommended today. I tend to beat myself up when I have disfluency issues. I'm always very hard on myself, but that is just the way I was trained. You have my permission to be kinder to yourself, as long as you also practice and work on improving your confidence.

My practice for public speaking on leadership and marketing is based on the methods I learned for slowing my speech and riding through the rough patches, so that I can be as fluent as possible. I tape-record my practice sessions, and if I hit a word that trips me up, I stop the tape and work on speaking through that roadblock until I master it. I also videotape my practices whenever possible, so I can play back each version and train my mind and body. Yes, body awareness and control are important for those who stutter, because your audience can pick up on your level of confidence—or lack of confidence—by observing your posture.

They won't want to watch or listen to your speech if your body language indicates that you are terrified, because that will make them uncomfortable too. Even your facial expressions are important, so when you videotape yourself, you can practice controlling them and keeping a so-called "straight face" during your speech. A happy face works too, and a big smile will do wonders for both you and the audience. Your facial expressions reflect your state of mind and the thoughts running through it, which is why you should work on your inner dialogue when preparing for a speech, too.

You see, what you tell yourself is every bit as important as what you tell your audience. You don't want to prepare for a speech or stand on the podium with negative thoughts racing through your brain, like runaway trains about to crash:

- *I'm terrible at giving speeches.*
- *My speech stinks.*
- *I'm about to ruin my career.*
- *People will be bored.*
- *I'm going to be so embarrassed.*
- *I'll die if I start stuttering.*

If you catch yourself thinking along these lines, hit the brakes. You aren't helping yourself with those negative thoughts. So, kick them out of your head. Visualize yourself giving them the boot, and replace them with more positive and helpful thoughts:

- *I've worked hard on this speech, and I'm ready to wow my audience.*
- *I've got this!*
- *They are going to love this speech! I'm sure of it.*
- *This will be so much fun. I can't wait for the standing ovation!*
- *Even if I stutter a little, I will power through the speech!*
- *My goal is to share my stories and information, just like a normal conversation.*
- *I am not on* American Idol, *so I shouldn't worry about being judged.*

The last one on that list is important, because some people go into a speech thinking about it as a performance with critics ready to pounce, or judges prepared to rate you. Remember, you aren't a contestant on a reality show—you aren't in a competition being judged by Blake Shelton or John Legend.

And don't feel that others are judging you either. Instead, focus on communicating with them, not performing for them. Think of your audience as friends and family members listening to you tell a story at a party. That mindset helps you stand at the speaker's podium with much less concern about being judged or rated by your audience.

Worth the Work

When it comes to public speaking, AIS experts recommend self-disclosure as a tool. If you step up to the podium and explain that you have a stutter, it can help you and the audience. You might even tell your audience that you won't let any stuttering bother you, so they, the audience, shouldn't let it bother them either.

Preparation is really the key to public speaking. If you know your speech inside and out, control your fears, and speak from the heart directly to your audience, you will be just fine up there. It takes some work, but it's worth it.

Having been the commencement speaker at the Fordham Gabelli School of Business and the Ohio State University Fisher College of Business in 2019, I encourage you to take a workshop on public speaking as I did, and then go out and *do* it! This is all about learning to manage fear, anxiety, and other emotions that we experience every time we have to speak. Just understand that these are quite natural feelings, experienced even by many people who do not stutter.

The fact is that once you get past your fear, actually delivering a speech can be much easier than you might expect. Many have learned that even if you have some fluency glitches while speaking, these tend to make the audience more attentive and the presentation more dramatic and interesting. That's an interesting approach and much different from the training I had, but if it works for you, go for it! The concept makes sense: Would you rather hear a speech from someone who is perfect and just drones on and on without any flair? How about someone whose presentation captures your full attention as you watch them overcome challenges, even as they speak to you?

One of the tenets of the AIS approach is to help those who stutter become comfortable with who they are and how they speak, which also helps others become more comfortable with them.

Working It Out

AIS and HCRI conduct many workshops across the country and around the year on public speaking for those who stutter. Those who go through their workshops often tell wonderful stories about the experience, which is designed to help them overcome their fear of public speaking by teaching them how to prepare, deliver the speech, and enjoy the process—free of crippling anxiety and fear. The graduates of these workshops often go on to join groups like Toastmasters or theater groups, because they've learned that public speaking can be therapeutic for them.

The workshops are group experiences in which participants support and encourage each other. They are taught how to organize their speeches with a beginning, middle, and end that flow well and are thus easier to deliver. Everyone gets to practice both prepared and impromptu speeches.

The instructors help participants understand that they don't have to be perfectly fluent to give a great speech or to be an effective communicator. They are taught body control methods, because so much of communication is nonverbal. Participants learn to control their response to moments of stuttering by maintaining eye contact and conveying confidence through their body language, so the audience is not distracted. The ultimate goal is to help those who stutter understand that what they have to say has value, just as they do, whether they speak perfectly or not.

Let me introduce you to an AIS workshop participant who benefitted from her experience. She is a delightful young lady with the wonderful name of Biibi Muse. As a seventeen-year-old high school student, Biibi described herself as someone with a covert stutter, but she realized that trying to deal with her fear of stuttering was wearing her out. She asked her school's speech therapist what she could do to get relief. After some research, the speech therapist recommended that she call the AIS satellite office that had just opened in Atlanta. Biibi eventually joined an intensive program for teens.

Carl Herder worked with Biibi, whom he described as having "a unique personality." She has learned to live more authentically, speak more freely, and be more open about her experiences with stuttering—to the point that she summoned the courage to deliver to the entire student body of her high school a "Slice of Life" speech about being someone who stuttered covertly.

Biibi graciously allowed me to share her speech with you, to demonstrate the powerful therapeutic effects of public speaking for people like us. She noted that she decided to give the speech because the workshop at AIS had helped her get rid of the feeling that her stutter was weighing her down. Giving the speech was a big step, but, she told Carl Herder, "When I took the thing that scared me the most and used it the way I wanted to, it changed everything."

Here then, is Biibi's speech, which I think you will find quite inspiring:

I will not talk about the things you think I am here to say. I will not talk about being Muslim or black or even a woman. I am here to talk about something I have tried to keep hidden for many years now. A part of myself I was in denial about for way too long.

For as long as I can remember, speaking was always a difficult thing for me, yet it may not be obvious due to the fact that I can't ever shut up.

Before this past year, speaking, specifically speaking fluently, was one of the hardest things for me. For years I tried to act in a way that I understood to be "normal."

I was the only kid I knew who stuttered and I felt as though it was something that needed to be hidden. I felt as though I had to hide my stutter because I thought stuttering made me stupid and that it was something that made people look down on me.

Because of this, I became a covert stutterer. As a covert stutterer, I did anything and everything possible to hide my stutter from everyone. From stomping my feet to slapping my thigh as I spoke, to analyzing every single word I could say. Stuttering controlled me more than I like to think it did.

Talking was always a burden for me, one that could not be avoided completely. For years I allowed myself to become caught up in my own head. I would think of every word I could possibly say and concentrate on the ones that I thought would lead to a stutter.

I knew that words that started with certain letters such as M, S, and O would most likely lead to a block, and I would try to change that word right before I said them.

Proper nouns had the same effect on me. I would try to avoid them by acting as though I couldn't remember it or giving a vague description. The constant act of processing and filtering out words became a norm for me. I could sift through words in my mind rather quickly or act as though I couldn't remember something to pass as fluent. This was better than being made fun of in my mind.

I did not realize how exhausting this was. I was constantly thinking of ways to hide my stutter and would always be on edge. Every conversation I had made me fearful because the thought of stuttering in front of another person was horrifying.

I felt as though I had no safe space. I was never really myself with anyone, including family and friends. For years, I attempted to be someone I knew I wasn't. I somehow developed the ability, in some situations, to speak for long periods of time without stuttering, so in my mind, I "cured" my stuttering.

For a couple of years, I went on like this, until my second semester of sophomore year, when all my tricks failed, all at once. I was left feeling isolated, and honestly, I thought I would never find a solution.

This took a huge toll on me mentally and it showed academically. I stopped participating in class and slowly began to just give up.

Once again, I felt like everything I wanted to do couldn't be done because of my stutter, and that this would inhibit me from being the person I've always imagined myself to be.

My stutter became too much to handle and I felt as though I had no one to help me. The idea of speaking out made me nauseous and I had no idea what to do next.

All seemed doomed until it was time to do a Spanish presentation. Stuttering is hard enough in English and with everything going on, I knew things were going to get ugly in class. Let's just say the presentation never happened and tears were shed later on.

Shout out to my partner though, because throughout that cringy process, they never made me feel as though I was stupid.

After that experience, I talked to my teacher and realized that it was time for a change. At this point, I was over keeping it hidden. I was fed up with the way I was making myself feel. I thought about it a lot and the thought of asking for help never crossed my mind until that very day.

I realized that it's okay to need help, and it's okay to need a lot of it. I thought, maybe I could be open about my stutter, at least with my teachers, and not take on all this alone. As things happen in high school, a new presentation was assigned in a different class, and as much as I would love to say I stood in front of the class and did my presentation without being afraid of stuttering, that didn't happen.

However, I did well on the presentation, despite me thinking that if I said something with a stutter it changes its value and means that what I said wasn't important.

For many people who stutter, the physical part of it is not the problem, it's mostly everything else, especially the reaction. I used to think that in order for something to be meaningful, it had to be said a certain way. This was big for me.

Never have I ever stood during a presentation and allowed myself to make eye contact during a block. Never have I told someone, specifically a teacher, that I stuttered and would need an accommodation. For the most part, I held myself back due to what I said.

I was so afraid of how people would react to my stutter, and to face the humiliation that came with that. I think what comes with getting older is realizing that some things are not in your control, and it's important to focus on what you can control. After that sliver of relief, there was no way I could go back. This teacher took it upon themselves to help me find help, and I am incredibly grateful for them.

Towards the end of the semester I was working with Danielle Moore to help find a way for me to get speech therapy, something I've never heard of for people who stutter. Thanks to Danielle's research, we found a company known as AIS, American Institute for Stuttering.

One of their speech pathologists had just moved to Atlanta. We stalked their website and watched some videos and decided to get into contact with them. Next thing I know, I'm signing up for a one week intensive with Carl Herder with three other boys and no warning as to what I was getting myself into. It's not called an intensive for nothing.

I don't know if it was because I was fasting and riding Marta and doing all this stuff, but it was one of the longest weeks of my life. I went from no speech therapy experience to a 10:00 am to 4:30 pm seven days a week where we did whatever Carl decided.

From phone calls to random restaurants to talking to strangers at Piedmont Park, the intensive was all about learning to accept your stutter and to learn to live with it.

The intensive course was all about speaking freely and saying what you want to actually say without all the negative thoughts. We debated, we talked, we laughed, and overall, we all were given a space where we could talk how we wanted, say what we wanted, in a room where everyone understood how difficult it is to do that on a daily basis.

At the end of the week, we invited friends and family to talk about what we learned in the intensive. Here's an excerpt from my speech back in June:

"Until this week, I always thought having a stutter was a negative aspect of my life. I kept it from friends, teachers, and even family members. Not only was I blocking in my speech, I began blocking a part of myself out. I decided that I will not let my stutter have that much control over me anymore. I am more than my stutter, and I have more to offer."

The week ended, and I was faced with the reality of what to do next. With most of my summer left, I began to talk about school and set goals for myself. I was able to point out the center *of my "onion diagram," those who I am most comfortable speaking with, and look at myself in a different light.*

I am not going to stand here today and say that I am completely done with my speech therapy or that I am completely confident in how I speak. I will say that I am working on accepting who I am, for how I am.

When the school year started, like most do, I understood the phrase "easier said than done." Aside from a small group of friends and family, no one knew I stuttered. Coming back to school meant coming back to a place where everyone thought I could speak fluent. It was hard.

Ninety-nine percent of what I dealt with had nothing to do with my stutter and more to do with everything else. The expectation we have around speech fluency and the negative stigma we attach to stuttering is one that is restrictive, and as a person with a stutter, it leaves me hopeless.

From a very young age, speaking fluently was always my number one goal because that was what society has as the norm. When I was not able to do that, I felt as though something was wrong with me, and that it was my job to change that. The reality of it is that I will most likely never speak fluent and that trying to hide my stutter only makes things worse for me.

One time in a session, Carl, my speech therapist said, "Stuttering is a communication disorder, not a speech disorder. Communicating things is a different mental process and it's different every time."

This means a lot of things obviously, but the main thing is that stuttering is dependent upon the stutterer. Some stutter more when reading something verbatim, like me, or stutter more in a conversation while they may read rather fluent.

What I do in speech therapy is most likely the exact opposite of what you think it is. We talk about ways to help me become a better speaker that stutters. We talk about how what I say matters, regardless of how it comes out of my mouth. I hope to convey that to you all now.

We are living in a time where teenagers are in a paradoxical standing, yet it is important for us to remember that we have more to offer than what people may first think.

As AIS says it, speak freely, live fearlessly. Thank you.

Key Points for Public Speaking

Thanks to Biibi for sharing her wonderful story. Her success is a great testimony to the power of public speaking for those of us who stutter. Here are a few other tips for stepping up to the podium and conquering your fears.

Remind yourself that you do not have to be perfectly fluent to make a great presentation. Perfection is for robots. You are not a robot.

Practice and practice your speech repeatedly so you are comfortable with it.

Record or videotape your practice speeches and play them back, especially those that you feel best about. Play back the best one before you go to bed the night before your speech.

Before your speech, visualize the audience members smiling, laughing in the right places, listening intently, and then giving you a standing ovation when you are done.

If you can arrange to check out the room where you will be speaking, go there and practice your speech and get comfortable in the space.

Control your breathing. Take deep breaths now and then to control your pace. If you feel yourself getting nervous, pause and take a couple deep breaths if that helps you. No need to rush!

Work out your nervousness with gestures, keeping that smile on your face and, if possible, walking around the stage as you speak. But take it slow and easy!

- Pauses can be your friend. Your audience won't mind!
- Even with a stutter you can be an effective communicator.
- In preparing and delivering a speech, use those methods that work best for you.
- Non-verbal communication is as important as verbal in giving a speech.
- If you seem comfortable with your stutter, your audience will be comfortable, too.
- Conveying confidence by maintaining eye contact and smiling helps you and your listeners.
- Do not worry about avoiding your stutter—go with it, and stay confident and composed.
- Remember, stuttering can make your speech more engaging for the audience.
- Accept yourself unconditionally and your audience will accept you, too.

9

Sing Your Song, Dance to Your Music, and Be Whoever You Want to Be

The wonderful actress Emily Blunt has had memorable roles in hit movies like *The Devil Wears Prada, The Girl on the Train, Mary Poppins Returns,* and *A Quiet Place,* but she may be an even bigger star at AIS—where she serves on the board with me and our other distinguished directors.

This beautiful, kind, and talented woman also has hosted many AIS events over the years, including our annual Freeing Voices, Changing Lives benefit gala. You see, Emily is one of us. She has a stutter, and an incredibly inspiring story of perseverance, resilience, and achievement to go with it—just like you and me.

But unlike most of us who stutter, Emily belongs to a fascinating group of individuals who found their own paths to greater self-confidence and fluency without professional assistance from speech-language therapists, speech pathologists, or trained clinicians. Emily's path was through acting.

Ed Sheeran's path was through singing. Jake Steinfeld's path was through fitness training and coaching under his "Body by Jake" brand. The late General Electric CEO Jack Welch found his path as a business executive, as did Home Depot co-founder Arthur Blank.

In fact, there are many, many others who are not celebrities or noted leaders who have built great lives by refusing to let their stutters define them. Instead, they have defined their own lives of accomplishment and achievement by making the most of their gifts instead of focusing on their stutters.

Dr. Grossman of AIS believes there are different pathways and methods for improving your speaking if you stutter. The majority of us find that the guidance of trained speech therapists helps us enormously. Yet some people say that, for whatever reasons, they could not find programs or guidance that worked for them. So instead, they managed to find their own way by tapping into special talents and skill sets that gave them the self-confidence, motivation, and inspiration from within.

One of these is the man with one of the most recognizable and wonderful voices in the entertainment world: James Earl Jones. After his Sunday school peers laughed at his stutter and teased him, Jones limited his speaking from first grade until his freshman year of high school, which he has identified as his mute years because he spoke only to his family and the animals on their Mississippi farm.

The distinguished voice that would grace *The Lion King, Star Wars,* and CNN was not heard publicly until a high school English teacher challenged him. The teacher thought a poem Jones submitted was so good, he couldn't believe Jones actually wrote it.

"I think you plagiarized it," Jones once recalled the teacher saying to him. "If you want to prove you wrote it, you stand in front of the class and recite it by memory."

Angry, Jones took the challenge and recited the poem to prove that it was his own. He did it without his usual bad stutter, and Jones realized that if he was reading or performing, he had much better fluency.

"I don't say I was 'cured,' I just work with it," he said in a National Public Radio interview.

Passion Overcomes Fear

While the name Lazaro Arbos may not be as recognized as Emily Blunt or James Earl Jones, this young man has a very similar story about rising above his stutter on a national stage. The Naples, Florida, resident was widely praised for doing that on the television show *American Idol*, during its twelfth season.

Lazaro dared to step up and sing in front of millions of people, despite the insecurities and fears he'd always felt because of his stutter. He didn't speak perfectly on the show during interviews, but that didn't stop him from performing his songs and earning praise from fans.

In this chapter, I want to share the stories of those who've found unconventional paths to greater fluency by pursuing their passions. I think you will find them inspiring, not because these people are famous or successful, but because, like you and me, they once felt alone, afraid, and frustrated because of their stutters—and yet, they found a path to a much better life than they'd ever imagined possible.

Many have never completely eliminated their fluency problems, but many have found that pursuing their passions has given them a greater purpose and helped them reduce their fears and insecurities. They've built confidence that has aided them in becoming better communicators and stronger people.

Singer Carly Simon is another example of this. As a child, her stutter frustrated her so much that when she couldn't get out the words "pass the salt" at the dinner table, she responded by singing them instead. The words flowed when she sang them, which was not the biggest surprise.

The real shocker was how everyone responded to her singing voice, which was beautiful. So in her case, stuttering led to the discovery of her great talent as a singer, which led to her eventually learning to thrive as a person who stuttered.

Researchers believe that those who stutter often can sing more freely than they can speak, because we don't feel as stressed and tense when we begin to sing. Additionally, when singing, we tend to prolong words more than when speaking. Some theorize also that individuals use the right side of their brain to sing to music instead of the left side, which is the area of the brain that controls language.

Speech pathologists and therapists have incorporated singing when working with other speech disorders, using methods including Melodic Intonation Therapy, which was part of Congresswoman Gabby Gifford's recovery program after she was shot and suffered traumatic brain injuries that made speaking difficult for her.

Most people who stutter can sing with fluency, which helps build their confidence in general. Singing and music treatments endorsed by the American Music Therapy Association are used to help those with autism, Parkinson's disease, and many other developmental and acquired disorders.

Speech therapists believe that music stimulates many areas of the brain, and that singing has a shared auditory-motor pathway with speech. The rhythms of music, singing, and rapping help provide cues that help with the timing and coordination of speech production. In addition, song lyrics are constant and unchanging unlike normal conversations, so singing can help alleviate the stress and anxiety for people who otherwise struggle with speaking.

Finding What Works for You

Most of us who stutter know the feelings of fear and frustration that accompany our speaking challenges and make it all the more difficult to communicate. Yet, some discover that in certain situations and settings, their fears, frustration, and the accompanying tension dissipate. They may have received training and assistance from professionals, but for whatever reason, they weren't able to find confidence and control of their voices until they discovered their own way to greater fluency. For some people this can occur while performing as an actor, singer, or dancer, or conducting business in an arena in which you feel supremely confident and knowledgeable.

"It isn't the activity that helps you with your speech pathways, it is learning that you aren't helpless and that you can have control and power over your voice that allays your fears. That can translate into your voice flowing more when you speak," Dr. Grossman told me.

Just as many of us who stutter have benefitted more than others from specific strategies, such as self-advertising, bouncing, or fluency shaping, there are those who, for whatever reasons—their mindsets or genetic makeup—seem to improve their fluency dramatically when they pursue their passions on stages or movie sets, in the gym, or in executive offices. On this phenomenon, Carl Herder of AIS told me:

> *This is a tricky thing to discuss when giving others advice. It's like they flip a switch and turn off their stuttering when they find a path that gives them greater self-confidence, and elevated feelings of competence and self-control. Finding her voice through acting worked for Emily Blunt and others, but it is not something we would design therapy around or make recommendations around. In many ways, it is a lucky happenstance that she and others have found their own therapeutic methods, but stuttering can be that way. You never know what might work for someone because every person and every stutter is unique.*

Acting It Out

Emily, who began stuttering around the age of seven, often says her parents had her try speech therapy, but it didn't seem to help her. Her speaking challenges seemed to get worse in adolescence. By the age of twelve, she was doing everything she could to avoid them. She felt an inner rage, because her stutter forced her to be someone other than the person she wanted to be.

"It felt like an emotional battle and a monumental mountain, like an imposter living within me," she once said at an AIS event.

Emily, who was born in a suburb of London, England, admired British poets and wrote poetry herself. She wanted to read it to her teachers, but she was terrified of stuttering. For the same reason, she despised being called on in her classes. As a teenage girl, she even avoided talking to friends on the phone. She was teased about her stutter by some classmates, whom she avoided as much as possible. If someone asked her name, she couldn't get it out.

"I was a smart kid, and had a lot to say, but I just couldn't say it. It would just haunt me," she told an interviewer for *W* magazine.

She struggled until one of her favorite teachers, Mr. McHale, whom she has described as an "enormous man with a massive mustache," asked her if she would like to be in the cast of a class play. Her mother had been an actress and her father was a criminal trial lawyer, which she thought of as acting too.

So, Emily was intrigued at the idea of being in the play, but she said no, because of her stutter. Again, "the imposter" behind Emily's fears and frustration forced her to avoid doing something she really thought she'd enjoy.

But then Mr. McHale did what great teachers so often do. He opened a door that his student had thought was closed to her.

"Emily, I've heard you doing silly voices and mimicking people, and you don't stutter when you do that, so why don't you use one of your other voices with an accent in the play?" he asked.

That was when the switch was flipped in Emily's life. She took the role, using what she now describes as a "very bad northern English accent," and it worked!

"Suddenly, I had a fluency," she recalled in a 2020 *Marie Claire* magazine interview. "And that was a very liberating thing for me as a kid. The removal of yourself from yourself, in some ways, was freeing."

From that first acting role, Emily realized that she could handle life and keep growing. Even at that point, though, she still had her sights set on going to college. She had discovered that, along with acting and using accents, she did not stutter when she spoke other languages. Her dream was to learn Spanish and work as an interpreter in the United Nations one day. She had come to feel that confident in her ability to communicate freely.

But when she went off to a boarding school called Hurtwood House in Surrey, England, she took a role in a rock musical called *Bliss* that was chosen for the Edinburgh Festival Fringe. One of her drama teachers at the school—the actor Adrian Rawlins, who plays Harry Potter's father in the movie series—thought she showed such promise that he recommended Emily to his agent, Roger Charteris.

Charteris signed her up as a client and began bringing her acting roles. The young woman who'd once dreaded speaking in class or on the telephone discovered that she'd fallen in love with performing. Along the way, Emily learned to love herself and her stutter, too.

The difference for her and for many AIS clients is that Emily no longer fears her stutter, nor is she ashamed of it. She now says that one of the things she loves about AIS is that they teach clients to accept their stutters as one of the things that make them unique and special.

Emily has come to realize that having a stutter helped her to become a very good listener, and more aware of the world around her.

"I was a really observant kid. I was a really empathetic kid and still feel that's something I try and lead with," she told her *Marie Claire* magazine interviewer.

The actress said she encourages empathy in her own children, so they embrace those who may be different from them, instead of teasing them.

Acting is the ultimate form of empathy, the actress added.

"You're empathizing with someone else's dilemma, with someone else's life, and so I think it frees you up. I just don't think anyone stutters when they're acting. So, I think you should try."

Living with a stutter also helped Emily realize that making mistakes is not a terrible thing, but a way to learn and grow—a lesson in being kind to yourself and others, she noted.

She still stutters occasionally, mostly when weary or when in an acting role requiring fast-paced dialogue, she said. But she no longer worries about her stutter when deciding which roles to take: "It is not something that I even think about. And any sort of stutter steps I might have, or things that I'll get tripped up on, or lines that could be tricky, I'll sort of just find a way around them. I think with experience, you discover the confidence in knowing you'll just find a way around it."

Like many AIS clients I've met, Emily has learned to take pride in her stutter.

"It's really not about, 'Oh, I stutter really badly.' It's more 'I stutter really well. I'm a brilliant stutterer,'" she said.

She encourages others who stutter to never feel like there is something wrong with them. "It's neurological, it's genetic, it's biological. It's not your fault. There's nothing you can do about it," she told her *Marie Claire* interviewer Sammy Blatstein, a young man who stutters and has spoken at AIS events.

Confidence Is a Key

Many of those who've overcome stuttering by pursuing a passion talk about how increased self-confidence has played a role in helping their speech fluency. A classic example of this is a true "self-made man," Jake Steinfeld, the pioneering "Body by Jake" fitness entrepreneur.

Jake worked with Hollywood celebrities including Steven Spielberg, Bette Midler, and Harrison Ford before launching his entrepreneurial career with his own line of health and fitness products. He has also created two fitness lifestyle networks, FitTV and ExerciseTV, and founded Major League Lacrosse.

Jake, who was part of the first class of AIS honorees to receive the Freeing Voices, Changing Lives award at our inaugural benefit gala in 2007, often talks about being an athletic but chunky kid who dreaded being called on in school because of his stutter. "When the teacher said we were each going to read out loud, I would rather have jumped off the Empire State Building," he recalled in an interview for the book.

If the teacher gave some warning ahead of time, Jake would try to memorize the reading assignment to help him overcome all the hurdles, which for him included the letters D, B, T, J, K, and L, among others.

When he hit a block on any of them, his stutter was so bad it "felt like [he] was drowning." Often, he'd hope the teacher would call on Laurie or Tommy first, two classmates who had worse stutters, so that by the time it was Jake's turn, "the other kids in the class would have stopped laughing and [he'd] sound like Maya Angelou compared to them."

Even today, despite all of his success and popularity, Jake recalls the anxiety he felt when forced to speak publicly.

"When we had Passover at our temple, you had to read aloud from the prayer book. Every family would do it together. I'd tell my father, 'Please don't pick me to read. Don't call on me.' Every now and then, I'd try to read, but I couldn't get through it," he said.

"Now, when I read from the prayer book as an adult, I always remember how hard it was back then, waiting my turn with the anxiety building up. Then, when my turn would come, everything would just start crashing and my stutter would spiral downward, getting worse and worse as I tried to hold on," Jake told me.

Like many of us who stutter, Jake developed avoidance methods to mask his problems with fluency. It didn't help that his elementary school in Long Island contacted his parents and suggested that they put Jake in special education classes.

"They wouldn't allow that to happen, but I never had any speech therapy classes either, if there were any offered back then," he recalled in our interview. "I struggled, even if it was just ordering a pizza on the phone, I couldn't do it. I'd hang up. You can't really understand what it's like if you've never stuttered. It's not the same as any other affliction. It can be crippling."

Jake was a fun-loving, outgoing kid who made friends easily, but he knew his fear of stuttering was holding him back. When he went to summer camp, the other kids called him "Typewriter" because they said he made a similar staccato sound when he stuttered. He hated being teased and laughed at.

Even as a teen, Jake had a lot of willpower. When he felt himself starting to withdraw from friends because of teasing and anxiousness over his stutter, he made the conscious decision to resist turning inward. The biggest boost came at the age of thirteen, when his father brought home a set of weights and Jake began working out in the basement on his own.

"As my body grew stronger, I realized I had more power over my life," he said. "The bigger my physique got the more I believed in myself. I saw myself as the underdog as opposed to a golden child. I liked it when people said you can't succeed because I wanted to prove them wrong, and prove to myself that I could do whatever I wanted to do with my life."

Now, lifting weights and building strength is not a cure for stuttering, but when Jake saw that he had the power to change his body in such a dramatic way, he began to feel that he could overcome any challenges in his life, including stuttering.

"When you build muscle, you stand up straighter and feel better about yourself and your power to control your life," he said. "I challenged myself to not stutter every day. Even though it was always there, and I'd always think about it, I learned to channel away my fears about it and even use it to my benefit."

His weightlifting and fitness regimen put Jake in position to become the pioneer of fitness training, and a very successful entrepreneur in the fitness and health industries. His exposure to high-powered executives and performers boosted his self-confidence and his ambitions.

Jake instinctively taught himself many of the basic techniques for overcoming stuttering that would become part of fluency shaping, avoidance reduction, and stuttering modification therapies.

"When I started to work with all these successful people, I learned to slow down and moderate my voice and inflection while controlling my breathing," he told me. "I always knew what I wanted to say, and by slowing down my speaking, I could avoid having the words fly out too fast and pile up like a train wreck."

Jake adjusts his tone and the pace of his speech to reduce his stutter when speaking in public, he said.

"I bring my voice down and make it slower, lower, and deeper. It's like an instrument that you learn to play," he said. "I discovered that when I go deeper with my voice, I don't stutter as much.

I really believe we all have our own ways of figuring out what works for us."

Jake, who lives by his motto, "Don't Quit!" worked out his own approaches to stuttering just as he had in his body-building sessions. His goal was always to define and control his own image, rather than letting anyone else define him.

He has been so successful at this that—along with making millions as an entrepreneur—Jake has often appeared in movies and television shows and even done voice-over for animated features including Disney's comedy *Ratatouille* and the drama *From up on Poppy Hill.*

"I've always created my own way to be myself in anything I've done," he said. "I made myself become very gregarious and outgoing instead of hiding my stutter. I learned to overcome the fear first. I trained my mind to say that it was okay even when I was scared. I told myself that I was going to get up and speak confidently until that monster in my mind got smaller and smaller."

We are all unique individuals, and we all have to find what works best for us in dealing with our stutter and the challenges that come with it. Jake, who still hits a block now and then, believes much of his success stems from the fact that he refused to be labeled as "the fat kid" or "the kid who stuttered." He was determined to create his own identity, and he has certainly done that.

As much as he tried to hide his stuttering when he was younger, Jake believes it made him an even stronger strongman. He will still self-advertise from time to time, and often talks about his stuttering. The funny thing is—many people refuse to believe him!

"I'll put it out there that I stutter when I tell the story of growing up and dealing with it, but a lot of times people will say, 'You're full of it, come on, Jake, I don't believe you ever stuttered!'"

Stronger Through Stuttering

Now, you may think it sounds crazy when a renowned health and fitness entrepreneur like Jake Steinfeld says that his stutter made him all the stronger, but he is not alone in feeling that way. This is not to diminish the fact that Jake and most others who stutter thought it was a burden when they were younger and had to endure teasing and anxiety.

Those feelings are shared by most of us who've had to deal with this challenge in our lives. Yet, like many other big challenges people face—whether it is a physical disability or a learning disorder of some kind—when we find ways to overcome and rise above them, we truly do feel like we've achieved something special. In turn, this makes us feel more self-confident that we can achieve our goals and our dreams. I've heard this time and again.

Another example of someone who feels this way about stuttering is Arthur Blank, the co-founder of Home Depot, who owns the Atlanta Falcons NFL team and the Atlanta United MLS team. In an AIS interview with Emily Blunt and another fitness trainer and expert who stuttered, Don Saladino, Arthur Blank talked about how he turned stuttering into a source of motivation.

"When I was younger, stuttering encouraged me to do more than I thought I could, and forced me to be more of myself and make sure if I had thoughts or feelings I was entitled to be heard," said the Harvard MBA graduate. "My mother encouraged me for sure, but I think it was wired within me, and stuttering gave me more of an incentive to do things in my life that I might not have done."

Arthur always encourages young people with stutters to be "true to your heart and purpose and be the best you can be."

"Fight through this, accept it as part of who you are, and learn to deal with it," he said. "Most importantly, know that your value as a human being and your contribution to society is not limited by whether you stutter or not."

Instead, Arthur noted, you set the limits for yourself according to the values you embrace and how you choose to live with or without them as your guidelines.

Don Saladino, who owns the Drive 495 gym in New York City where clients including Ryan Reynolds, Blake Lively, and Hugh Jackman have worked out, said even though he was teased about his stutter from the second grade on, he would never change that part of his life. In the end, it motivated him to be better and do better.

"It seemed like a disability when I was young, but now when I try to influence people positively, if I stutter I don't do retakes or delete the video. I am proud of it," he said.

I hope you've been inspired by these stories from those who've found unique paths to managing their stutters and rising above them to pursue their passions. As someone who has worked on improving my speech fluency throughout my life, I can also tell you that there are great benefits to be found in modern therapy programs as well.

The most important thing is that you understand your stutter does not limit or define your success. There are many paths to a better life open to you.

10

The Power of Community for Those Who Stutter

Ross Horton struggled with stuttering from the age of three. He was twenty-eight years old before he fully realized that he was not alone in those struggles and, in fact, that there was a world of support and understanding out there for him in the global community serving those who stutter.

Ross discovered that world when his mother encouraged him to attend a conference of the National Stuttering Association. She even offered to join him if he'd agree to go. Like many of us who stutter, Ross had often felt isolated by his communication challenges, and he saw no reason to hang out with other people who shared them.

So, at first, he rejected his mother's idea, but then he thought, "It's time. You need to do this. It will be worth it," he wrote in a 2019 article for *Letting Go*, the online newsletter of the National Stuttering Association.

And the trip *was* worth it—even more than Ross had ever dreamed it would be. For the first time in his life Ross discovered a welcoming community of support and understanding, at the NSA's 2019 annual conference in Fort Lauderdale, Florida.

Shortly after Ross entered the Marriott Harbor Beach Resort where the convention was being held, another attendee introduced himself and asked Ross's name. He admits in the article that he freaked out a little and struggled to get his name out. But then, Ross found himself surrounded by sympathetic, encouraging, and helpful strangers.

"It was as if an emergency response team had just gathered around me—and they all knew exactly how I felt," he wrote.

It's going to be all right, buddy. Take your time!

Stutter like a rock star, Ross!

No fear here, we're all the same.

Ross had locked up in his attempts to speak many, many times before, but never before had he felt that he wasn't alone in his life-long struggle to speak freely.

"It was an incredible feeling to finally be able to identify with others who completely accepted and understood me and my stutter," he wrote in the *Letting Go* article.

That is the power of the many support groups, social media pages, websites, and other communities that serve people who stutter around the world. Most speech therapists and pathologists believe that group therapy is an effective approach for reducing avoidance behaviors and treating the emotional aspects of stuttering that form the "hidden" part of the iceberg. Usually there are no more than six participants in the groups at AIS, where they meet once a week for an hour and a half.

These sessions work on helping clients achieve their individual goals and objectives. They practice speech skills, engage in discussions, and do assignments. The discussions focus on strategies for dealing with fears, shame, and embarrassment in daily life.

Clients are provided with methods for creating and following weekly plans when they are home. They receive feedback on their progress toward their goals. The AIS approach provides them with models of new behaviors, explanations, and resources, as well as written treatment plans and progress reports.

Support groups and organizations also are an important part of the recovery process and daily lives of many of us who stutter. I have a go-to person myself. For me, it's Holly Humphreys at HCRI. When I'm having a difficult day with my speech, I call her for advice. The call really helps.

"We encourage just about all of our clients to join groups and organizations for those who stutter as part of their therapy," Carl Herder told me. "For most people it is a really important part of the stuttering treatment."

Carl noted that the motto for the National Stuttering Association is "You are not alone," which is a powerful message when you grow up feeling misunderstood and disconnected socially. Whether you attend local meetings and events, national conventions, or online chats, bonding with others who stutter and sharing information, experiences, and feelings, can be life-changing on many levels.

The NSA, which has more than two hundred local support groups in the U.S., provides information, increases public awareness, serves as a referral for resources, offers support to professionals in the field, and advocates for the stuttering community. They also hold workshops and a national convention that brings together all who stutter and those who support them.

As Ross Horton discovered, when you meet so many others who share your experiences and have walked the same path, you suddenly feel like you are part of something greater than yourself. You feel safe to speak freely.

"Many people go to these meetings and realize they've been holding back in sharing their feelings, experiences, and opinions," Carl told me.

He noted that while most of his clients have benefitted from joining organizations for those who stutter, there are some who aren't ready for such an immersive experience into that community.

"The caveat is that some people do not like support groups because they say it's like looking into a mirror and they don't like what they see," the speech-language therapist told me. "But sometimes I've asked clients who haven't enjoyed these meetings to try them again because it might take a couple visits before you find people you can bond with and have a better experience."

One of Carl's clients was shaken after attending his first NSA conference in Texas because he felt like after being around so many others who stuttered, his own was more prevalent than ever. The AIS speech-language pathologist urged him to go back, and that client eventually became an NSA chapter leader.

"Stuttering is complex and sometimes being around people who stutter can be really beneficial," he told me. "But for some, it can also stir things up. Usually in hindsight they feel it stirs things up in a good way, though it doesn't always feel that way in the moment."

Others report that they find that attending events for those who stutter is like a breath of fresh air, but some need more of an acclimation period, the speech-language therapist said.

Coming Together

We think it's wonderful to have a sense of shared purpose and to support and encourage each other.

You may still be searching for a circle of friends who stutter; if so, I certainly encourage you to do so. I would also urge you to join larger organizations that support and advocate for those who stutter. I understand that not everyone is "a joiner," and some people are more outgoing than others. Just know that there are big communities and smaller groups available throughout the country and around the world.

If you can't find one near you through your work, your speech therapist, or any other way, don't be afraid to start your own. I know many people who have done that over the years. Some have struggled to organize at first, but most eventually find that there are many others out there searching for people to connect with who have similar challenges.

Jai Prakash "J.P." Sunda, who became coordinator for the national Indian Stammering Association, told Peter Reitzes of *StutterTalk* in a 2012 interview that he struggled to start his first local group in India for those who stutter, like him. After several unsuccessful efforts to find a speech therapist who could help him, J.P. decided to put together a group of people who could help each other. He'd belonged to a speech therapy group as a teenager and found it helpful, so he thought it might work even better for him as an adult, he said.

"I learned that if there was a bunch of people who stammer and understand the problem, it was helpful for me to practice and experiment with my speech," he recalled in the *StutterTalk* interview. "I never thought I could stammer openly. I never thought stuttering was even allowed, but that group gave me a nice feeling where you were more at peace."

At first J.P. thought it was "absurd" to even consider starting his own group because he'd struggled with fluency shaping and thought only someone who had become 100 percent fluent would have the credibility to do that.

"I thought people might judge me on my stuttering and say, 'Since you haven't cured yourself, how do you plan to help others?'" he said. "I thought they wouldn't take me seriously."

Eventually, though, the pain of his loneliness and isolation compelled him to try and recruit others who stutter for a group. Initially, a speech therapist gave him a list of potential contacts, but none of them responded to his emails. He then tried creating a post to put on the bulletin board of the company where he worked in IT.

"It took me a whole day to post it because I thought people would think negatively of me," he said in the *StutterTalk* interview.

Finally, J.P. found the courage to post the sign looking for others who stuttered. Then, one week passed. No responses.

"Two or three weeks later, I only got one response from another colleague who stammered, and we decided to meet every week. But he never showed up."

To his credit, J.P. did not give up. He tracked down contact information from others who stuttered and began calling them. This time, he told a small fib to make them feel more at ease about getting together.

"I told them I already had started a self-help group, with two members," he said.

For some reason, that worked, and about a half dozen people showed up for the first meeting. They began meeting regularly and grew from there, giving J.P. the confidence to later become the coordinator for the national stammering organization in his native country.

"Being vulnerable is hard, and sometimes people are not that motivated to show up and talk about the thing that they struggle with the most in life," said Carl. "It can be a lot of hard work to organize and manage a group, but it can be really wonderful too."

FRIENDS You Might Like

AIS Director Dr. Grossman and Los Angeles social worker and stutter therapist Nora O'Connor are among the many fellow professionals who support the organization FRIENDS: The National Association of Young People Who Stutter, a national non-profit.

FRIENDS is led by co-founder Lee Caggiano, a speech-language pathologist whose son stutters. Each year they host an annual convention, as well as many regional one-day conferences for young people who stutter and their families.

The conferences encourage discussions in a group setting where it is okay to stutter, and where stuttering is accepted by all who attend. Teens who attend often make comments such as this one: "It was so nice just to be me today."

The success of the FRIENDS conferences has proven that those who stutter and their families find great benefit in having places where they can help connect with others facing the same challenges. That was one of the conclusions of a 2016 *StutterTalk* episode hosted by author and NSA member Reuben Schuff, an aerospace engineer and advocate for people who stutter. His guests were clinical social worker Nora O'Connor and speech-language pathologist Loryn McGill of California, who coordinate and design the Southern California FRIENDS conferences.

The *StutterTalk* guests and host noted that family members often come away from such meetings with completely different perspectives on stuttering and how to help their loved ones who stutter. They also benefit from being in a group where it is okay to stutter and to talk about stuttering.

Loryn McGill shared that there have been life-changing moments at the end of each FRIENDS conference when participants, who often feel isolated and alone in their challenges, talk about their experiences in a final session. At one of those sessions, a family gave an emotional presentation on accepting their son and learning to look beyond his stutter. The audience was in tears because you could see the impact it had on them, according to those present.

Another person who attended the conference for the first time said, "I think my life would be much different if I'd done this a long time ago."

The speech therapists said that organizations, groups, and gatherings for those who stutter can be an essential part of their treatment. Having a supportive community will help younger generations understand that even with a stutter they can communicate well and build fulfilling and accomplished lives.

"There is so much power in the community that gathers," said the *StutterTalk* host.

"It's one thing to tell a child, 'There is nothing wrong with you,' but to get them in front of a couple hundred people to give this same message has more impact than you can ever get in a one-on-one session," noted Loryn McGill.

Parents benefit from attending FRIENDS conferences and other gatherings, too, because it often changes their view of stuttering, how it impacts their children, and how they can best help their children deal with this complex challenge.

Power In Numbers

Emily Blunt has often noted in her AIS appearances and speeches that an encouraging community of support is extremely important for others who stutter because there is value in knowing that others are going through the same experiences.

Carl of AIS shared these suggestions on how to build a sense of community and support.

1. Go online and search for stuttering organizations.
2. Check the campus organization listings at local colleges and universities.
3. Look for local chapters of the National Stuttering Association.
4. Check social media, like Facebook, for stuttering group pages.
5. Listen to *StutterTalk* and other podcasts related to stuttering and for those who stutter.
6. The International Stuttering Association has a helpful website with very good articles and guidance, including a resource page for starting and operating a stuttering group. The ISA also hosts an International Stuttering Awareness Day conference each year.

Stutter Social

Another big proponent of support groups and networking for people who stutter is Mitchell Trichon, who has a master's and PhD studying speech-language pathology with a focus on stuttering. He is a co-founder with David Resnick of Stutter Social, an organization that uses web-based video conferencing and a smart phone application to provide support to people from over fifty countries.

Stutter Social is a support group that connects those who stutter through Google+ Hangouts (group video chats). In the Hangouts, participants share similar stories, laugh about tense feelings, learn about speech techniques, and build self-acceptance. Its membership community is international, with participants from countries including the United States, Canada, Mexico, England, Scotland, France, Croatia, India, and New Zealand.

There are four weekly Hangouts and occasional special guest Hangouts. Stutter Social also promotes awareness and understanding of stuttering to the public. Their website is http:// stuttersocial.com.

Mitch has helped to lead a national network of over one hundred adult support groups. He serves on the faculty at La Salle University in Philadelphia, where he conducts research on self-help activities for people who stutter.

Here is a list of stuttering support groups, organizations, blogs, and websites that can also provide valuable information and a sense of community.

- The American Institute for Stuttering
  www.stutteringtreatment.org
- Hollins Communications Research Institute
  www.stuttering.org

- The National Stuttering Association
  www.westutter.org
- American Board of Fluency and Fluency Disorders
  www.stutteringspecialists.org
- American Speech-Language-Hearing Association
  www.asha.org
- A Free Voice
  www.afreevoice.org
- British Stammering Association
  www.stamma.org
- Canadian Stuttering Association
  www.stutter.ca
- FRIENDS: The National Association of Young People Who Stutter
  www.friendswhostutter.org
- International Stuttering Association
  www.isastutter.org
- *Make Room for the Stuttering* Blog
  www.stutterrockstar.com
- Passing Twice: A Place for LGBTQ People Who Stutter and Their Allies
  www.passingtwice.org
- Say: The Stuttering Association for the Young
  www.say.org
- Stuttering Foundation of America
  www.stutteringhelp.org
- *StutterTalk*
  www.stuttertalk.com

11

For Parents: Helping Your Child Fight the Gremlins

My mother's daily advice to "work harder and be smarter" to overcome the handicap of my stutter stayed with me throughout my life. She inspired me to excel in my career and in my efforts to communicate effectively, despite my significant stuttering challenges.

I am well aware, then, of just how important it is for parents to encourage and support children who stutter. Kids who stutter have more frustrations and insecurities to deal with than most, but they should never be made to feel inferior, not as smart, or less loved than other children.

This chapter, then, is for the parents and loved ones of people who stutter. My goal is to help them understand the "stuttering gremlins" that mess with our minds, stirring up negative and self-defeating thoughts and emotions that make it even more difficult for us to speak.

Dr. Grossman talks to parents and their children about the stuttering "gremlins" that can make those who stutter retreat from their daily communications and activities to avoid potentially unpleasant situations. She describes them as toxic creatures, including the negative inner voice that can lead to self-defeating decisions.

In a 2018 article on the AIS website, she notes that these negative thoughts are rooted in a collection of hurtful experiences, such as encounters with bullying, teasing, or embarrassment because of a stuttering moment. She described stuttering gremlins as "destructive creatures of the mind who spew forth a collection of unhelpful thoughts that, when obeyed, seem to afford safety from potentially painful speaking situations."

In reality, though, listening to their chatter results in an influx of negative emotions, resulting in tense, avoidant speech behaviors, Dr. Grossman added. For example, if a person enters a situation worried that he will be mocked for stuttering, he will speak with more anxiety and a more severe physical struggle during his attempts at avoidance.

"These inner gremlins send strong messages to the child who stutters that he should try hard to *not* stutter, that he should avoid talking when he thinks he will stutter a lot, and that others will think badly of him when they notice it," she wrote. "In short, the gremlins scream: 'Don't stutter! It is *not ok!*'"

Dr. Grossman said stuttering gremlins want us to accept negative feelings about stuttering without question, in an effort to "squelch your vibrancy and joy for living."

The gremlin may pose as something that can protect you and your feelings, but in reality, it often leads young people astray. They try to hide their stutters, and as a result, they tend to hide from life itself—including the best parts of life.

Dr. Grossman also wrote that your gremlin would coax you to worry incessantly about things you cannot control, to relive your past mistakes over and over again, and to feel anxious about the future.

Don't let the gremlins get to your children. Encourage them to listen to their hearts and find their voices. Tell them to speak freely even if they do stutter. Help them fight off fear, anxiety, and discouragement. One day, they will thank you for helping them find their voices.

Parents and their loved ones must help guard their children against these stuttering gremlins because they send strong negative messages, making them think they should try hard to *not* stutter, that they should avoid talking when they think they may stutter a lot, and that others will think badly of them.

Dr. Grossman—as well as the majority of therapists in the field—believe that the most important goal for children is to keep them speaking freely, regardless of how they are presently stuttering. To help you do that, they have shared with me three methods to help parents and other caregivers squash the gremlins that try to stifle children's voices.

Three Methods to Help Parents and Caregivers

1. Introduce Children to Role Models Who Stutter

When you are young and you stutter, you tend to think that no one else in the world has it as hard as you do. That is how I felt when I was bullied and laughed at. And I didn't want to be around anyone else who stuttered, because they only reminded me of how others must perceive me. What really helped me was learning that there were successful and famous adults who stuttered. Knowing that famous public figures like Sir Winston Churchill, television host Jack Paar, and even Marilyn Monroe stuttered helped me see that there was a path forward for me.

Parents today can go online and find videos of modern-day celebrities—ones I've mentioned throughout this book, like Emily Blunt, Bruce Willis, and Ed Sheeran—talking about how they too once felt alone and unpopular because of their stutters. By introducing your children to others who stutter in person and online, you can help them see for themselves that people who stutter can become excellent communicators, as well as successful, popular, and empowered to be whatever they want to be in life.

There are many videos featuring those who stutter on the AIS website that you can share with your children. You can go to the AIS website and do a search for them: www.stutteringtreatment.org.

Here are just a few people featured in those videos that Dr. Grossman believes could help your child:

- Ziauddin Yousafzai, the Pakistani education activist whose daughter Malala was awarded the Nobel Peace Prize for championing the rights of young women.
- George Springer, an outfielder for the Houston Astros Major League Baseball team.
- Emily Blunt, the actress and AIS board member.
- Regular people and AIS clients Jolie and Joshua.

2. Encourage Your Children to Say What They Want to Say, Even If They Stutter

Dr. Grossman and the other therapists at AIS believe that your child should feel free to speak, rather than try to avoid stuttering.

Most people find this liberating, and in the end, they find they can speak more freely if they have this mindset.

Parents can promote this approach by being active listeners, keeping normal eye contact with their children as they speak, and not putting time pressure on them. It will also help if you reinforce the power of the child's message, not the level of fluency. Praise your children as superheroes for being brave enough to face stuttering head-on.

3. Teach Your Children to Be Their Own Friends and Advocates

Children who stutter often may be more compassionate to others than they are to themselves. Dr. Grossman says it is helpful to promote the idea that just because someone "notices" something, this does not mean it is judged as "bad." After all, we notice when people have foreign accents or if they are very tall, and those are not bad things at all. They are just different.

You may find it helpful also to encourage your children to roleplay to help them figure out the most useful ways to respond when someone asks them about their stuttering or comments on it. Parents can also spare their child embarrassment by teaching them to recognize when someone is asking out of kindness and curiosity, or setting them up for criticism.

We further emphasize teaching children to self-disclose their stuttering to others by saying something like, "I stutter, so it may take a few extra seconds for me to talk, but don't worry, I'll get there." This can help alleviate negative stuttering anticipation and time pressure.

The AIS therapists teach children that their true friends will be there to support them no matter what, and that those who would bully them are the ones to be pitied and ignored. To make this point, they quote Dr. Seuss, who said, "Those who mind don't matter, and those who matter don't mind."

It is worth emphasizing again that parents and family members should encourage children to speak freely, without worrying about their stutter. This is easy to say, but not so easy to do, I know; unfortunately, experts say that the fear of stuttering just piles challenges on top of challenges for the child.

The emotional burden heightens anxieties and tension, which make communication even more difficult. This is why children adapt avoidance behaviors. They don't want to be hurt so they avoid words that trigger their stutter, or they avoid speaking as much as possible. Concerns about provoking negative reactions and teasing from schoolmates also tend to result in unconscious body movements and avoidance of eye contact, which further complicate their efforts to fit in and interact with peers.

Dealing with Parental Fears

The parents of children who stutter shouldn't neglect their own emotional and mental well-being. You have a right to be concerned, but don't get caught up in "worst-case scenario" thinking or become so overwrought that your child can sense something is wrong and feel like a burden on you.

Former AIS board member Jake "Body by Jake" Steinfeld, whose stuttering challenges were featured earlier in the book, makes this point when explaining his reaction to hearing his daughter stutter at a young age.

"When Morgan was born, we thought she was the smartest kid in the world—like all our kids," he recalled. "Then when she first started talking, she was chirping away like you wouldn't believe. But one day, I was driving her to pre-school in the car and she was in the back in her car seat when she said, 'D-d-d-d-dad…' and I'll never forget, my heart started beating because I was so worried that she might have a stutter like me."

Jake's concerns—and guilt—only grew when Morgan continued to stutter regularly over the next five days.

"This is worrying me. I can't believe I've given this to my daughter. We need to call somebody and help her," Jake told his wife Tracey.

She gave Jake a look and said, "Why are you so worried? You have a stutter and you turned out okay!"

Still, Tracey went along with Jake's plan to call a speech pathologist to discuss what they should do if Morgan's stuttering continued. In the first few minutes, Tracey wondered if she should have taken Jake to a psychiatrist instead.

"I was flipping out," he admitted. "I told the speech therapist that Morgan was stuttering and that I had stuttered, and I was worried if it was contagious. I was freaking out and saying things that people had said about me when I stuttered as a kid."

The speech therapist tried to calm Jake.

"Let me ask you some things," she said. "When you are with your daughter, do you ask her a lot of questions like, 'How are you doing?' and 'What is going on?' And when she gets in the car after school, do you ask her how her day went? Or if she met any new friends?"

The therapist went on: "And when you have friends over, do you ask Morgan questions so you can show off how smart she is?"

Jake answered yes to all of the therapist's questions about his questions.

The expert then offered this therapeutic approach for Jake.

"Here is what I want you to do, Mr. Steinfeld: *Shut up!* Do not ask your daughter any more questions. You can talk to her and tell her things, but don't ask her questions, please. She is just six years old and this is a very normal thing, and in most cases, her stutter will go away soon if you don't keep asking her questions all the time."

Jake realized that because he loved his daughter and wanted to know what was going on in her life, he "was barraging her with questions and her young brain couldn't keep up."

Once Jake stopped the daily interrogations, Morgan's stuttering went away. Now, as we all know too well, this isn't always the way things play out. The point is that parents often can do more harm than good, even if their intentions are pure. So, if you have concerns—and as soon as you have concerns—don't be afraid to talk to a speech therapist or anyone with expertise on children who stutter.

Find out what you can do to help your child feel loved, self-confident, and deserving of the best life has to offer, whether the stutter goes away or stays. Here are a few other basic tips for parents and family members of those who stutter:

- Try not to speak in a hurried way to your child.
- Make sure all family members take turns talking when you are together.
- Avoid using long, complex sentences or jargon that your child might not understand.
- If your child stutters, do not interrupt or say the word for them or tell them to "spit it out." This includes telling the child to "take your time" or to stop and take a breath.

- Just be a good and patient listener, and repeat their words to them so they understand that you heard and processed what was said.
- Communicate with your child using a good balance of comments and questions, not just questions (as Jake said he was doing with his daughter).

The Unexpected Gifts of Stuttering

I thought I'd end this chapter for parents with an inspiring story they can share with their children. This is the story of Nolan Russo Jr., who has stuttered since early childhood and still stutters occasionally today. In many ways, Nolan's story is similar to those of all of us who have been accompanied by stutters on our life journeys. Yet, I wanted to share it with you because of my friend's interesting perspective on his stutter, and how his feelings about it have changed since he was a child.

So, please keep in mind Nolan Russo Jr.'s story when your child struggles with stuttering, and please, encourage your child to speak freely, without fear.

Most parents of children who stutter can identify with the concern that Nolan Russo's mother, Linda, felt when she noticed his disfluency early on. "As a mother you see your child struggling and you feel his struggling and frustration and his pain, and you feel helpless," she said.

Fortunately, Mrs. Russo and her husband, Nolan Russo Sr., brought their son to AIS at a young age, and the speech therapists there helped him manage and rise above his stuttering challenges. "It changed my life," he said.

Today, Nolan Russo Jr. is CEO of Capital Printing in Middle-sex, New Jersey. He also serves as the treasurer of the AIS Board of Directors and has served in the past as the board's chairman.

My friend eventually realized the burden that had plagued him since childhood as a source of unexpected gifts. He spoke about those gifts in a speech given at the 13th Annual AIS Gala in 2019, when he was the honoree. These quotes are from his speech transcript.

"I'm in fourth grade, I'm ten years old transferring schools. I don't know anyone, and nobody knows me," he said. "First day of school, the teacher wants to introduce me. She gestures for me to introduce myself to the class, to everyone. I always stuttered saying my name, so I stand up. Panic takes over. I force myself to the front of the class, and I say 'Hi my name is No-No-No.'"

"I have a bad block and can't get it out. A kid in a front row seat hadn't been paying much attention. He says under his breath, 'What, did you forget your name?' The teacher didn't hear him, but I heard him. Next to him, his buddy says, 'I think he said his name is No-No-Nobody.' Nice to meet you Nobody!"

All of us who stutter have been through that humiliation and taunting. There is no escaping it. Nolan recalled how the next day, he was looking forward to gym class because he was good in sports, but again his stutter tripped him up.

The gym teacher was organizing baseball teams and he asked Nolan what position he wanted to play. Nolan loved to play third base, but when he tried to tell the teacher that, he hit a block and couldn't get it out. The gym teacher impatiently passed over him and sent the other nine remaining kids out to the field, leaving Nolan as the only one on the bench. He recalls the teacher saying he'd put him in when Nolan could decide what position he wanted to play. The boy knew what position he wanted to play, just as he knew his own name. His stutter had prevented Nolan from saying what he wanted to say, and being who he wanted to be, once again.

"And that is what stuttering does to you," he said. "It takes away your ability to express yourself. You are like two people; the person who stutters and the other person who is trapped inside."

We all feel isolated when this happens. We feel alone, depressed, and frustrated just like Nolan. His parents saw this and tried to find help for him. They enrolled him in programs to alleviate stuttering during his grammar school years, but their methods didn't seem to help him once he left the clinic—and he didn't like the message they seem to send.

"The problem was they approached stuttering like, 'Something is wrong, and we are going to fix it.' Like something is broken with you and we are going to fix it and you can't be yourself or the person you want to be until we fix it," he recalled.

Then, when Nolan was fourteen, his parents learned of the therapeutic approach to stuttering created by the founder of AIS, the late Catherine Otto Montgomery. They enrolled him in the three-week intensive program over the summer. After his previous experiences with stuttering programs, he was not hopeful when his parents told him.

"I went in as a stutterer desperate for relief," he recalled in his passionate talk. But he'd come to believe that he was broken and couldn't be fixed.

Just a few days into the AIS program, however, Nolan realized "something profound and important," he said.

"Their approach was unlike anything I had ever experienced. It is subtle but so profound…you are not a stutterer at AIS. You are a person who stutters. You might think that is just simple semantics, but the difference is I was a person who stuttered, I was a person who had brown hair and I was a person who was good at athletics and a person who was smart and funny and whatever you want to put in that blank spot."

The message that Nolan took into his heart was that his stuttering did not define him or limit his life in any way. In fact, he began to understand that in many ways, stuttering had made him a stronger person.

"My stuttering made me a more compassionate person. I respect peoples' insecurities and don't take advantage of it. It made me more insightful. I couldn't dance around with words. I couldn't engage in BS. I had to be direct and honest in my responses. My words were a valuable currency to me, I couldn't just waste them. It made me more courageous, more hardworking, and more resilient."

Nolan no longer felt broken, or in need of fixing, he said.

"I was exactly who I needed to be: me, a person who stuttered. And that is empowering. That acceptance is empowering, and oh, by the way, fluency follows that acceptance. I know that at AIS fluency is not the goal, but inherently when you form a different relationship with your stutter that changes," he said.

For most of his life, Nolan had felt ashamed and guilty for stuttering, but his speech therapists helped him see it in a new light: "as a source of strength that makes you unique and gives you an advantage, and it is empowering," he said.

"I'm thanking you not as a guy standing behind the podium, but as a ten-year-old kid standing in front of that class," my friend said in concluding his moving speech.

Nolan Russo's life will never again be limited by his stutter, and that is something every parent of a child who stutters should see as a pathway to better days.

12

Words of Caution, Encouragement, and Inspiration

As someone who has stuttered for most of his life, I've found and heard some wonderful advice, therapies, and treatments. I've also come across some truly horrendous advice, and unhelpful—even damaging—treatments. This is a common experience.

Before I send you off to the world to speak freely and live fearlessly, I want to caution you to be careful about buying into any programs, therapies, or treatments that claim to "cure" stuttering. There is no sure cure out there—at least not yet.

Just last year, in 2018, the alarms went off for me and my friends who are professional speech therapists and speech pathologists after we watched an episode of the television talk show *Steve*.

The host Steve Harvey likes to give advice on all sorts of matters, even those that may not be in his wheelhouse, to put it kindly. He may have meant well when he offered advice to a young woman who stuttered on this particular episode, but some of the guidance he offered raised concerns among professionals who have devoted their lives to helping those with stutters.

The talk show host made the claim that stuttering is "curable" and that there is nothing "physically" wrong with anyone who stutters. It's true that some people do stop stuttering permanently, but, as noted earlier, there is no universal sure cure that works for everyone. And there are definitely neurological, genetic links to stuttering, so it is not merely a psychological problem, as Harvey's comments seem to suggest.

He also made the troubling claim that stuttering therapies are largely unhelpful, and speech pathologists who do not stutter themselves do not understand it. To put out an umbrella statement like that is not helpful.

Believe me, I know there are effective therapies and truly helpful speech therapists out there, just as I know there are some quacks and poseurs who make false and misleading claims and do not have adequate training.

You need to be cautious, and even skeptical, when searching the internet for help with your stuttering. You should not ever pay for treatments without checking out the program thoroughly, which includes speaking to individuals who've been treated successfully.

When you search for a speech therapist, make sure you find one who does have training and experience working with those who stutter, because, as Dr. Grossman tells me, "Stuttering treatment is very different than working with other problems."

She noted that there are currently fewer than two hundred speech-language pathologists who are certified as specialists in fluency by the American Speech–Language–Hearing Association.

Many speech therapists who treat stuttering do not have specialized training.

Your best sources of information and guidance are those organizations and individuals who are dedicated to helping those who stutter, and also those who have found treatments and professionals who've been helpful.

On his show, Steve Harvey offered several more bits of advice that most professionals who work with people who stutter would not recommend. He also told the young person with a stutter to rehearse her responses three times in her head before verbalizing them. This is a strategy that actually can backfire and increase tension for us, according to most experts.

I'm not condemning Steve Harvey. I'm sure he meant well, but he was offering guidance outside of his area of expertise as a talk show host. You want to deal with experts. And you want to avoid those who are merely trying to make money off of those seeking help.

Be cautious about where you look for answers and treatments for stuttering. There are many questionable characters who advertise online, on television, and in print media. Some claim or suggest that surefire cures are available through hypnosis, yoga, meditation, herbs, essential oils, diet plans, and both prescription and over-the-counter medications.

While many of these treatments may help promote healthier lifestyles in general and reduce anxieties that can exacerbate stuttering, they are not cures by any means. Certain medications can be helpful, but there are no FDA-approved medications for symptomatic treatment of stuttering. Self-medication is always a slippery slope. You should always seek the advice of your doctor and professionals before going down that path.

My Journey

Finally, I wanted to share with you a bit more of my personal journey as someone who stutters. It began as a kid growing up in Brooklyn, New York. At an early age, my first nemesis was an unlikely one: a popular cartoon character beloved by many.

I don't know who I hated more—that character, Porky Pig, or the guy who created him. If you are not familiar with Porky, he is known for his severe stutter. He appeared in hundreds of cartoons, and was often featured in the final moments, offering his signature line: "Th-th-th-that's all, folks!"

Younger generations may know Porky mostly from more recent appearances in the *Space Jam* movies, and *The Looney Tunes Show* on Cartoon Network, but he's been around since the 1930s and is rated as one of the top fifty cartoon characters in history.

I remember going to the Commodore Theatre on Sunday afternoon with my friends for an action-packed double feature—a John Wayne war movie and a Hopalong Cassidy western. These were usually separated by a Walter Lantz cartoon.

I prayed the cartoon wouldn't show Porky Pig, but since he was the big moneymaker of the Walter Lantz film studio in the 40s and 50s, it definitely did. For many, he was a beloved character. But when I heard him stutter away, I wanted to crawl under my seat. I felt the eyes of my buddies peering at me, sharing my embarrassment and horror at the way Porky painfully stuttered.

My friends didn't laugh—but the other movie patrons sure howled every time Porky's face turned red, trying to get a word out! Like most of you in this room, stuttering was never funny to me.

Little boys can be cruel, and some big boys could be even crueler about stuttering. My nose has been broken three times. It happened twice as a kid, when I was fighting someone who had made fun of me, and then later in the army, when I took on a pretty mean guy who was a lot bigger than me. The good news is, the army guy never ridiculed my speech again. The bad news was…my nose was black and blue for a week and still

Looks terrible!

I hated the fact that stuttering was one "life obstacle" I could not fix easily. I decided early on, even after going through every kind of speech therapy program known to man (my mom was not a quitter), that this was *not* going to be a handicap for me. I could not permit my stuttering to be an impediment to my personal aspirations. Most days I handled it well, but not always.

I remember at the age of fifteen going out with this beautiful cheerleader from Midwood High School in the center of Brooklyn. I was the envy of all of my friends. She was a knockout! But one day I phoned her to confirm our Friday night date and she said, "Wow, you know, the wallpaper hanger was over today and he spoke just like you. He couldn't get a word out."

I hung up, and that was the last time we spoke.

Was that the smartest approach? It's easy to say now that I could have helped her understand how hurtful her comment was. But at the time I felt as if I had been gut-punched. It took me a while to recover. I expect that many of you have had similar experiences.

My life with a stutter has been an adventure, to say the least. I needed to leave Brooklyn, and at the age of sixteen and a half, I was off to Columbus, Ohio, as a freshman at the Ohio State University—with a goal of winning a spot on the college baseball team. That was a challenge!

They recruited the best baseball team ever that year, and I got cut after pitching my third pre-season game. Without a hoped-for scholarship, I worked a zillion different jobs in order to stay out in Columbus, because I loved the Ohio State experience so much.

After graduation, I enlisted in the U.S. Army, where I was fortunate to become a speechwriter for General Earl C. Bergquist. The general took a liking to me. And then, because of that fortuitous experience, I later worked as a junior speechwriter for President Kennedy's brother Bobby when he ran for the Senate in 1964.

When Bobby Kennedy won, I wanted to go to Washington; however, personal circumstances prevented that from happening. I found myself in need of a job and the pharmaceutical industry beckoned. I started in public affairs with a company called Lederle Laboratories in Pearl River, New York. It was later acquired by another pharmaceutical company called Wyeth in 1994, which was purchased subsequently by Pfizer in 2009.

Elevating My Game

After a few years, I became bored with public affairs, and so I used the G.I. Bill to go to graduate school at Fairleigh Dickinson Graduate Business School. I had to keep my day job, so I went to school at night and on the weekends until I finally got my MBA. Then, came the luck of a person who stutterers, the dean of Fairleigh Dickinson decided to write the president of Lederle to let him know that one of his employees was the MBA valedictorian.

Two weeks later, I was placed in the company's management development program, where I had a ball. After being shuffled from department to department for training, I ended up in marketing—where I had wanted to be all along.

I put my nose to the grindstone and began working my way up through the ranks. First a product manager, then a group product director. But then, for reasons I couldn't understand, after I was running the company's most successful divisions, the promotions came to a halt and less successful people began moving past me.

After running into brick walls with my boss and human resources, and not being able to get any kind of a straight answer as to why I wasn't being moved up to general manager (the position I wanted), I took a call from an executive recruiter.

A small advertising agency in New York wanted a new CEO. I took the job, and, without a bit of sadness, I left Lederle, the company I had cherished for eighteen years. I settled into that job; later that year, on a snowy Christmas Eve, a former member of the Lederle management board asked me out to lunch.

I cancelled my holiday plans and agreed to meet him at a Chinese restaurant on Route 59 in Nanuet, New York, called Hong Luck. I remember as if it was yesterday. This wonderful person, who had resigned from the company shortly after I left, explained, "Sander, I have prostate cancer. I don't know how long I'm going to last. I want you to know why I resigned from the executive committee."

He then told me that when my name had come up for promotion two years before, an influential member of the committee said, "We can't promote Sander to general manager. Stuttering is a form of mental illness."

This idiot then proceeded to convince two other members of the executive committee of this specious notion. My luncheon companion, who passed away six months after that Christmas Eve in 1984, attempted to change the vote…but without success.

So now, I really could see the "glass ceiling" I had faced. At that point, I had a choice. On one hand, I could feel sorry for myself and furious at the idiot who sabotaged my career. I could become spiteful, hateful, angry, depressed—you name it.

Or I could simply move on. It was a *crucible experience* and moving on seemed like a much better choice, and so, I did.

Finding My Voice

During this time, my speech and dysfluencies improved dramatically. In 1978, as you've read by now, I attended the HCRI in Roanoke, Virginia. I was fluent for the first time in my life and God, what a difference it made. I finally felt that I had the fluency targets to hold onto, and that if I practiced them religiously—which of course is almost impossible to do—I could be fluent most of the time, and in some cases, all the time. But of course, we never seem to practice enough and keep going back to "spontaneous" fluency, which, for stutterers, is the absolute pits.

So, while I have some great days and some not-so-great days, I'm still a big fan of the Hollins program and Dr. Webster, as well as AIS. I constantly encourage people to think about AIS and Hollins as ways to improve their fluency.

But, as I've said, some days are a lot better than others. I do a lot of public speaking: a lot of interviews, a lot of presentations, some TV, and even a weekly radio show on PSR. Isn't it amazing how fluent you are when you're on TV and need to act?

Today I'm a lot older, a little wiser—but the issues are still the same. And the biggest issue is: Are you going to feel sorry for yourself when you have a painful speech day? Are you going to become depressed, beat yourself up, and say, "Why me?"

Or will you continue to move on and work a little harder to be smarter than the competition? Are you ready to focus on your strengths and be fearless in facing the world?

As I noted earlier, for years I taught a lecture class at Fordham University Graduate School of Business. I always made a point on the first day of class to say to my students—many who considered English their second language—that, in fact, I am a stutterer and I will have dysfluencies.

I told them it's OK to *not* have perfect speech or speak in perfect English. It doesn't make any difference. My point to them, and what I really care about, is *what* they have to say rather than *how* they say it.

My hope for you is that the world of work has become more understanding and kinder to those who stutter than it was back in my day. Let's hope that today's top management, particularly the Gen-Xers, have a more informed and gentler approach.

I am hopeful, too, that one benefit of being in the new and more diverse global economy is that people are much more accepting of speech differences, including stuttering.

As I noted, my stuttering will always be the *crucible experience,* which will always keep me sharp and prepared to do whatever I do next, usually to a level that rises beyond expectations. I have found that those who stutter are often perfectionists, never quitting until they excel at whatever they do.

I have seen this with inspiring people I've met through my advocacy on behalf of stutterers—most of whom I've mentioned in this book—including the late General Electric CEO Jack Welch, Home Depot co-founder Arthur Blank, Vice President Joe Biden, broadcaster John Stossel, actors Bruce Willis and Emily Blunt, and singer-songwriter Carly Simon.

They work on their speaking every day—and so can we all.

I hope you have found this book helpful and inspiring. Finally, let me leave you with this message: "There are those who fall but get back up, who lose but don't accept loss, and who succeed because they refuse to fail. These people don't teach by words, they inspire by example."

I hope this book has inspired you as much as all of those who stutter inspire me in their quest to create lives of fulfillment and accomplishment.

—*Sander A. Flaum*

ACKNOWLEDGMENTS

There are some amazing people who helped me with this book for those who stutter and their families.

Wes Smith, my collaborator on this book, was a wonderful partner and a fantastic writer.

My assistant for the past twenty years, Lisa Pollione, was there for me on this project, as always.

Dr. Heather Grossman and her team of speech therapists as well as Dr. Ron Webster made incredible contributions to this book. I want to also single out AIS speech-language pathologist Carl Herder for his helpful observations.

Also, my fellow friends who stutter including Jake Steinfeld and those on the AIS committee—Eric Dinallo, Nolan Russo, Susan Jensen, and John Stossel—for their insights and great stories about their lives.

Bridget Chapman, speech therapist and coordinator of the Flaum Fluency Program, and chairperson of the Department of Speech and Hearing Science at the Ohio State University, Dr. Robert Fox, who built the stuttering fluency program with the assistance of JoAnn Donohue.

Arthur Blank, co-founder of Home Depot, owner of the Atlanta Falcons, and a staunch supporter of AIS, who helped build their Atlanta-based office.

Many thanks to Shannon Marven, head of Dupree Miller, for her wisdom and advice, and to Anthony Ziccardi, for his wise counsel as head of Post Hill Press.

Christine Madden, the planner and producer of the AIS Annual Gala.

Finally, to my two beautiful children Pamela Weinberg and Jonathon Flaum, my lovely sister Adele, and my wonderful cousin Dr. Stan Kissel, for their continuing love and support.

BIBLIOGRAPHY

American Institute for Stuttering. "Emily Blunt Discusses Stuttering with Arthur Blank and Don Saladino–AIS Gala 2019." 2019 American Institute for Stuttering Gala. July 31, 2019. YouTube video, 10:23. https://www.youtube.com/watch?v=gxVVxB7eKN8.

American Institute for Stuttering. "Speech Therapy." Accessed September 1, 2020. https://stutteringtreatment.org//speech-therapy.

Beilby, Janet M., Michelle L. Byrnes, and J. Scott Yaruss. (2012). "Acceptance and Commitment Therapy for Adults Who Stutter: Psychosocial Adjustment and Speech Fluency." *Journal of Fluency Disorders* 37 (4): 289-99. https://pubmed.ncbi.nlm.nih.gov/23218212/.

Blatstein, Sammy. "How Emily Blunt's Stutter Led Her to a Successful Acting Career." *Marie Claire*, February 11, 2020. https://www.marieclaire.com/celebrity/a30729273/emily-blunt-stutter-interview-2020/.

Brocklehurst, Paul. "Mindfulness and Stuttering: How Can Mindfulness Help?" Stammering Self-Empowerment Programme. Accessed August 20, 2020. http://www.stammeringresearch.org/mindfulness.pdf.

Campbell, Patrick, Christopher Constantino, and Sam Simpson, eds. *Stammering Pride and Prejudice: Difference Not Defect* (Surrey, UK: J & R Press Ltd, 2019).

Constantino, Christopher. "Stuttering Gain." International Stuttering Association. Accessed August 20, 2020. http://isad.isastutter.org/isad-2016/papers-presented-by-2016/stories-and-experiences-with-stuttering-by-pws/stuttering-gain-christopher-constantino/#_ftn1.

D'Agostino, Sarah. "Who Is George Daquila?" *Letting Go*, Spring 2016. https://westutter.org/wp-content/uploads/2016/11/Spring-2016-FINAL.compressed.pdf.

Dinallo, Eric. "Facing the Fear of Stuttering." 2017 American Institute for Stuttering Gala. August 2, 2017. YouTube video, 8:23. https://stutteringtreatment. org/portfolio-items/eric-dinallo-facing-fear-stuttering-2017-ais-gala/.

Dinallo, Eric. "The Moment Every Adult Stutterer Dreads." *Atlantic*, December 8, 2019. https://www.theatlantic.com/ideas/archive/2019/12/feeling-every -adult-stutterer-knows/603220/.

Dmitriy. "Being a Teacher Who Stutters." American Institute for Stuttering. March 11, 2013. https://stutteringtreatment.org/being-a-teacher-who -stutters/.

Dmitriy. "How AIS Helped to Free My Voice and Change My Life." American Institute for Stuttering. March 4, 2015. https://stutteringtreatment.org/ how-ais-helped-to-free-my-voice-and-change-my-life/.

Gennuso, Sam. "4 Things to Know about Recovery from Shame." American Institute for Stuttering. January 30, 2020. https://stutteringtreatment.org/ recovery-from-shame/.

Goldstein, Chaya. "My Journey Home." American Institute for Stuttering. January 26, 2018. https://stutteringtreatment.org/my-journey-home/.

Goldstein, Chaya. "Self-Advocacy in the Workplace: 4 Tips with George Daquila." American Institute for Stuttering. February 13, 2019. https:// stutteringtreatment.org/self-advocacy-in-the-workplace/.

Green Sheehan, Joseph. *Stuttering: Research and Therapy* (New York: Harper & Row, 1970).

Grossman, Heather. "Helping Children Squash Their Stuttering Gremlins." American Institute for Stuttering. October 30, 2018. https://stuttering-treatment.org/helping-children-squash-their-stuttering-gremlins/.

Grossman, Heather. "Response to Steve Harvey's Comments about Stuttering." American Institute for Stuttering. October 16, 2018. https://stuttering-treatment.org/response-to-steve-harveys-comments-about-stuttering/.

Grossman, Heather and Gunars Neiders. "Holistic Approach to Stuttering Using Rational Emotive Behavior Therapy." International Stuttering Association. Accessed August 20, 2020. https://isad.isastutter. org/isad-2016/papers-presented-by-2016/research-therapy-and-support/ holistic-approach-to-stuttering-using-rational-emotive-behavior-thera-py-heather-grossman-gunars-neiders/.

Hartley, Sarah. "James Earl Jones: My Stutter Was So Bad I Barely Spoke to Anyone for Eight Years." *Daily Mail*, March 6, 2010. https://www.dailymail.co.uk/health/article-1255955/James-Earl-Jones-My-stutter-bad-I-barely-spoke-years.html.

Herder, Carl. "AIS Honoree Ed Sheeran 2015 Gala Speech." American Institute for Stuttering. June 11, 2015. https://stutteringtreatment.org/ais-honoree-ed-sheeran-2015-gala-speech/.

Herder, Carl. "Meditation Resources to Help in Your Stuttering Journey." American Institute for Stuttering. May 2, 2017. https://stutteringtreatment.org/meditation-resources/.

Horton, Ross. "A First Time for Everything." *Letting Go*, Fall 2019. https://westutter.org/wp-content/uploads/lg-fall-2019.pdf.

"Intensive Stuttering Therapy: Rose and Carl Talk about Stuttering Modification Strategies." March 8, 2019. YouTube video, 4:17. https://stutteringtreatment.org/portfolio-items/intensive-stuttering-therapy-rose-carl-talk-stuttering-modification-strategies/.

Leiman, Brooke. "The 411 on Voluntary Stuttering." *The Stuttering Source* (blog). September 21, 2013. http://www.stutteringsource.com/blog/the-411-on-voluntary-stuttering#.XwzFRi2ZOis.

Mertz, Pamela A. "About Me." *Make Room for the Stuttering* (blog). Accessed August 20, 2020. https://stutterrockstar.com/who-am-i/.

Moisse, Katie, Bob Woodruff, James Hill, and Lana Zak. "Gabby Giffords: Finding Words through Song." ABC News, November 8, 2011. https://abcnews.go.com/Health/w_MindBodyNews/gabby-giffords-finding-voice-music-therapy/story?id=14903987.

"Nolan Russo Honored by the American Institute for Stuttering." 2019 American Institute for Stuttering Gala. July 31, 2019. YouTube video, 10:26. https://stutteringtreatment.org/portfolio-items/nolan-russo-gala-honoree-speech/.

O'Connor, Nora. "Self-Image Issues." Minnesota State University, Mankato. Accessed August 20, 2020. https://www.mnsu.edu/comdis/isad5/papers/women.html#oconnor.html.

O'Connor, Nora, Loryn McGill, and Reuben Schuff. "'It Was Just So Nice to Be Me Today' (Ep. 572)." March 20, 2016. *StutterTalk*. Podcast, 23:18. https://stuttertalk.com/tag/nora-oconnor/.

Peim, Benjamin. "The Promising Research behind Mindfulness and Stuttering." *Meditation* (blog). Headspace, accessed August 20, 2020. https://www.headspace.com/blog/2017/02/04/mindfulness-and-stuttering/.

"Putting it Bluntly." *W Magazine*, October 1, 2007. https://www.wmagazine.com/story/emily-blunt/.

Reitzes, Peter. "The Why and the How of Voluntary Stuttering." Minnesota State University, Mankato. July 18, 2005. https://www.mnsu.edu/comdis/isad8/papers/reitzes8.html.

Reitzes, Peter and Jai Prakash Sunda. "Stuttering Modification: Melting the Fears Away with Jai Prakash Sunda (324)." March 11, 2012. *StutterTalk*. Podcast, 51:35. https://stuttertalk.com/stuttering-modification-melting-the-fears-away-with-jai-prakash-sunda-324/.

Smith, Morgan and Mary Green. "How Emily Blunt Overcame a Childhood Stutter—and Helps Others Do the Same." *People*, March 4, 2020. https://people.com/movies/how-emily-blunt-overcame-a-childhood-stutter-and-helps-others-do-the-same/.

Stuttering Foundation of America. "James Earl Jones." Accessed August 20, 2020. https://www.stutteringhelp.org/famous-people/james-earl-jones.

Stuttering Foundation of America. "John Stossel." Accessed August 20, 2020. https://www.stutteringhelp.org/famous-people/john-stossel.

Stuttering Foundation of America. "Samuel L. Jackson." April 29, 2015. https://www.stutteringhelp.org/content/samuel-l-jackson.

Sullenberger III, Chesley B. "Capt. 'Sully' Sullenberger: Like Joe Biden, I Once Stuttered, Too. I Dare You to Mock Me." *New York Times*, January 18, 2020. https://www.nytimes.com/2020/01/18/opinion/sully-biden-stutter-lara-trump.html.

Sullivan, Kate and Eric Bradner. "Biden Opens Up about Stuttering and Offers Advice to Young People Who Stutter." CNN, February 5, 2020. https://www.cnn.com/2020/02/05/politics/joe-biden-stutter/index.html.

Tsaousides, Theo. "Why Are We Scared of Public Speaking?" *Psychology Today*, November 27, 2017. https://www.psychologytoday.com/us/blog/smashing-the-brainblocks/201711/why-are-we-scared-public-speaking.

Wartofsky, Alona. "Dark Side of the Actor Harvey Keitel, Plumbing the Depths of the Soul." *Washington Post*, September 13, 1995. https://www.washingtonpost.com/archive/lifestyle/1995/09/13/dark-side-of-the-actor-harvey-keitel-plumbing-the-depths-of-the-soul/2d7c6a94-43ba-4f32-983c-d1c8657ae70a/.